Childbirth doesn't have to hurt

About the Authors

Nikki Bradford is an award-winning medical author and respected health journalist. She has been Health Editor and consultant on several national women's magazines, including *Good Housekeeping* and *Essentials*, and has written 12 other bestselling titles, including *The Well Woman's Self Help Directory*, *Men's Health Matters* and *The Miraculous World of Your Unborn Baby* and *The Hamlyn Encyclopedia of Complementary Medicine*. Nikki is an associate member of The Royal Society of Medicine, and founding honorary secretary of The Guild of Health Writers. She has two children, Ben and Jessie.

Dr Geoffrey Chamberlain is currently Professor of the History of Medicine in Wales, and has written or contributed to more than 500 clinical research papers and 50 books on pregnancy and childbirth, many of which have become essential educational texts for medical students. He is a former president of the Royal College of Obstetricians & Gynaecologists, and a former editor of the *British Journal of Obstetrics & Gynaecology*.

Childbirth
doesn't have
to hurt

Nikki Bradford
Professor Geoffrey Chamberlain

Expert Advisory Panel

I am deeply grateful to the following people, all of whom are leading experts in their fields, for their invaluable help, generous professional advice and enthusiasm for the book.

On this new and fully updated edition:

Prof Geoffrey Chamberlain
Geraldine O'Connell, Professor of Obstetric
 Anaesthesia at St Thomas' Hospital, London
Dr Michel Odent, Director of the Primal Health
 Foundation, and water birth pioneer
Sarah Budd, Head of the Acupuncture Midwifery Team
 at the Royal Devon and Exeter Hospital, and
 Assistant at the Acupuncture Research Centre, Exeter
 University
Dr Alice Green, former Chairwoman of the British
 Autogenic Training Society
Dr David Chamberlain, past President of the
 International Association for Pre- and Perinatal
 Psychology & Health, San Diego, USA

On the first edition of this book, published in 1995 (all titles relate to the consultant's positions at the time of publication):

Orthodox medicine

Felicity Reynolds, Professor of Obstetric Anaesthesia,
 St Thomas' Hospital, London
Dr David Bogod, Secretary of the Obstetric
 Anaesthetists Association

The Royal College of Midwives, especially President
  Caroline Flint
Nicholas Fisk, Professor of Obstetrics & Gynaecology
  at Queen Charlotte's Hospital, London

Natural methods

Rowena Davies, Head of Midwifery Services, and the
  midwifery team at St George's Hospital, London
Acupuncture Christina McCausland, acupuncturist and
  co-founder of Acupuncture for Childbirth
Aromatherapy Dr Vivian N Lunny, aromatherapist,
  former pathologist, and currently Head of Research
  for the scientific committee of the Aromatherapy
  Organisations Council
Autogenic Training Dr Alice Green, homeopath, GP
  with the Diploma in Obstetrics, and Vice President
  of the British Autogenic Training Society
Breathing & Relaxation Helen Lewison, Chairwoman
  of The National Childbirth Trust
Homeopathy Barbara Cummins, homeopath and
  midwife
Hypnotherapy Dr Les Brann, GP and hypnotherapist
Massage Stephen Sandler of the British School of
  Osteopathy, and Consultant Osteopath at the
  Portland Hospital for Women & Children, London
Reflexology Farah Begum Baig, reflexologist and
  Director of the Hope Clinic, Cambridge
Water Janet Balaskas, Founder of the Active Birth
  Movement and Director of the Active Birth Centre,
  London

ISBN 1-84333-617-0

A catalogue record for this book is available
from the British Library

First published in 2002 by
Vega
64 Brewery Road
London, N7 9NT

A member of **Chrysalis** Books plc

Visit our website at www.chrysalisbooks.co.uk

Printed in Wales
by CPD

Contents

Introduction

Having a baby? Want some good news? Childbirth doesn't have to hurt. There, we've said it – and it's true.

There are more than 20 methods of pain relief available to women in the West – from epidurals and 'gas and air' to acupuncture and homeopathy – and this book lays out the facts and figures behind every one of them.

Together with advice from your obstetrician and midwife, *Childbirth Doesn't Have to Hurt* will help you make an informed decision about which method of pain relief will suit you best, so that you can bring your baby into the world in the way that you want – and he or she deserves.

The Labour Process

Labour is the powerful process by which babies are usually brought into the world. It involves your womb contracting to make itself smaller and open up its exit so your baby can go through and pass down your vagina to be born. One obstetrician describes it as 'the day your baby's first home becomes his launch-pad'. Some babies are born by Caesarean on an operating table, some at home on a beanbag, some under water, and some on a bed. Whichever way your baby arrives, the following pages give you detailed information about the different stages your labour will pass through so that you will know exactly what is happening at every moment – and why.

When Labour Begins

Towards the end of their pregnancy, many women have had enough and just want their baby to come out. Their expanding size is making them increasingly uncomfortable, and any problems that may have developed earlier in their pregnancy, such as backache, tiredness, piles or varicose veins, will probably get worse in the final few weeks.

The popular image of a pregnant woman glowing with health, sitting peacefully with her hands folded over her rounded, neat belly is a myth. And unfortunately it's a persistent one that still manages to make many mothers feel bad when pregnancy is not like that for them. In reality, many find that their abdomen has apparently dropped down to their knees, and that they feel lethargic and irritable most of the time. And as their baby's head becomes more firmly engaged, even walking may become uncomfortable, leaving women counting the days until their delivery date.

Many midwives suggest that this feeling of, 'Right, I've had enough now, I just want that baby out so I can meet

D-Day
Remember the expected due date you were given early in pregnancy? Your baby probably won't arrive on it – only one in 20 babies does. So it's worth having a due week or fortnight in mind instead.

Which day?
More babies are born on Wednesdays and Thursdays than on any other day of the week. The least likely days for them to arrive are Saturday and Sunday.

him or her' is useful biologically and psychologically, as it helps prime women for the major effort of labour itself.

Key dates and times

About 90% of babies are born between 38 and 41 weeks after the first day of their mother's last menstrual period. About 5% are 'late', defined by doctors, midwives and obstetricians as after 42 weeks. All these arrival zones are normal. Some 6% are born 'early', before 38 weeks.

Labour has three main stages, and together they usually last six to 24 hours. The average for first births is seven to nine hours, and for subsequent births four to five hours.

What happens first?

People tend to treat a heavily pregnant woman with great caution, as if she is an unexploded bomb, likely to detonate at any minute. But they don't need to. General lifting (perhaps of a toddler or bags of shopping), walking extensively, making love, and even bumps and minor falls are unlikely to cause labour to start if your body and your baby are not ready for it.

The latest research suggests that it's probably your baby who starts labour off. As he begins to run out of room inside you and perhaps gets less food and oxygen, he will become a little stressed and begin to release hormones. These cross the placenta into your own bloodstream. Once in your system they encourage your body to make more hormones – the ones that start your womb contracting.

Your labour could begin in any one of several ways. Early signs include:

■ Regular contractions of your womb that come and go, and which become painful after a while.

■ The loss of some bloodstained discharge from your vagina. Called the 'show', this is the plug of mucus that has been sealing off your cervix, or the neck of your womb, protecting your unborn baby above. It becomes dislodged when your cervix starts opening in preparation for the birth.

■ Your waters break.

When your waters break

This happens when the membranes of the amniotic sac, which keeps your baby surrounded in warm fluid, rupture. It doesn't hurt, but some women feel a distinct 'popping' or 'pinging' sensation. If your waters break you may not necessarily be in labour – some women's waters leak or break several weeks before they go into labour (a small early leak may repair itself). But always let your midwife or doctor know if it does happen. And yes, contrary to what mothers used to be told, it is safe to have a bath if your waters have broken as long as the bath itself is very clean.

When the amniotic sac breaks open, it may do so with a sizeable tear or a small split. Depending on where the membranes have broken, you can experience your waters breaking either as a quick gush of fluid, or a discreet, intermittent trickle.

If the break in the membrane sac is at the bottom of the womb near your cervix, you will probably feel a gush. If it is further up, your baby's head will act as a partial plug, stopping the fluid rushing out, and you will only feel a trickle that stops and starts. When waters break as a trickle, women often worry that they have wet themselves, but the amniotic fluid has a very distinctive scent, which is not a bit unpleasant and nothing like that of urine. You will easily be able to tell the difference.

Your waters can break as much as a day or two before labour begins. For a few mothers, it may even be several weeks before, in which case they would have to be admitted to hospital to help prevent a premature labour. As to the most usual time of day – there isn't one. People often say that the most common time for it to happen is when you are in bed at night, but this is probably because you are in bed for eight hours at a time, the longest period you are likely to be in one place in a day.

Many women become worried that their waters will break somewhere public, and embarrassing, like a business meeting if you are working up till the last moment, in the cinema, or at the supermarket (one national chain even used to offer to pay for all the shopping the mother

A trickle not a tidal wave
When your waters break it may feel like a great gush of fluid, but it is usually only between two tablespoons and a cupful.

It's not like the movies

The classic image of a woman's waters breaking dramatically when she starts labour is a bit misleading. It only happens that way for about one in 10 women, though it's more usual in mothers who have had a baby before.

had in her trolley if this ever happened in one of their stores). Yet it is no more likely to occur when you are out and about than it is at any other time. If you are concerned about this you could always wear a highly absorbent incontinence pad (like a sanitary towel) when you go out. You can get these from any chemist. If you are worried that your mattress may get wet, you may like to place a rubber undersheet beneath the bottom sheet halfway down the bed. Or cut open a large bin liner and use that instead.

If you lose what appears to be a large amount of fluid do not worry that you will have what some people call a 'dry labour'. More fluid is being made by the lining of your womb all the time, so the amount you will have inside you after another few hours should not be affected by what you lose.

The breaking of your waters can often make your contractions more powerful and speed up labour, sometimes quite dramatically. This is partly because the baby's head can press more directly against your cervix if it is no longer cushioned by the sac of amniotic fluid, and this produces an increase in oxytocin, the powerful hormone that causes your womb to contract. It may also be that the sac membranes themselves contain a hormone that encourages

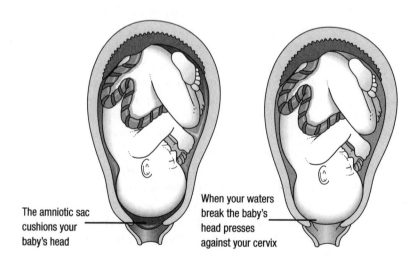

The amniotic sac cushions your baby's head

When your waters break the baby's head presses against your cervix your womb to contract and that this hormone is released when they rupture.

Other indications

Early on in labour you may also feel period-like pains, a low backache, abdominal cramps, pains down the inside of your thighs, in your hips and even in your knees, and pain and discomfort in your rectum (back passage) that feels like constipation. If you are having your baby at home, ring and tell your midwife if any of these symptoms (or anything unusual) occurs. If you are having your baby in hospital, phone the labour ward and talk to the midwife on duty. Depending on the symptoms you describe to her, she will either suggest you come in to hospital or that you stay at home for a few more hours.

'I thought I just had indigestion, but it wasn't stomach ache – I was in labour'

Although contractions, the show, and your waters breaking can all suggest that labour has begun, none guarantees that it has definitely done so. It is sometimes difficult to tell for sure. It is easy, for instance, to mistake strong and regular Braxton Hicks contractions (p20) towards the end of pregnancy for those you feel in the first stage of labour. And if this is your first baby, you have nothing to compare what you are feeling with. If you've had a child before, you will usually find that your body moves into labour more smoothly for subsequent births and that the entire process is easier. Many women say that it is as if their body just remembered what to do right from the beginning.

False labour

Sometimes women have false labours, where their contractions begin but then fade away. This can happen at intervals for a couple of weeks before labour really begins. False labour is caused by your womb flexing to slowly manoeuvre your baby's head into the right position deep in the lower part of the pelvis. The good thing about this is that it is usually a run-up to the real thing and, frustrating though it can be, at least it tells you that your baby's birth is now very near.

Braxton Hicks contractions

False labour isn't the only time you may have practice contractions. Most women notice their womb hardening at intervals throughout their later pregnancy. These are practice squeezes called Braxton Hicks contractions. While they don't usually feel uncomfortable, they may be strong enough to make you catch your breath or stop still for a moment. More often than not, though, they will be mild enough for you to continue whatever you are doing.

Understanding the differences between these practice squeezes and genuine labour contractions will help you know whether you are really in labour yet or not.

Braxton Hicks contractions:
- Do not become closer together over time. They remain irregular, showing no sign of forming a pattern.
- Stay the same strength throughout, before dying away.
- May be a bit uncomfortable but are not particularly painful.

Labour contractions:
- Become steadily stronger over time.
- Come more and more often, and form a pattern.
- Start gently, build up to a peak of intensity, then die away each time.
- Definitely feel uncomfortable or painful.

What is a contraction?

A contraction is when the muscles of your womb are working very hard. Womb muscles are remarkable pieces of bio-engineering, and are made quite differently from other muscle masses. They are laid down in a series of spirals of about two turns each. Each muscle spiral has a mirror image of itself, so that a pull on the left-hand spiral combined with a similar pull on its right-hand counterpart gradually reduces the size of your womb.

Unlike other muscles in your body, the muscle fibres of your womb become slightly shorter and fatter each time they contract. Because the muscles do not revert to their former size after they have finished contracting, the overall effect is that after each contraction your womb gets a little bit smaller.

Your contractions may be uncomfortable and even become downright painful later on, but they are doing four vital jobs to help you get your baby born:
■ They are making your baby's first home gradually smaller so that he is encouraged to leave it.
■ They are helping to position your baby for birth. With each contraction, your womb axis tilts slightly forward to encourage your baby's head into the right position so that it can enter your birth canal.
■ They help pull up and dilate (open) your cervix until it has flattened out and become wide open.
■ They push your baby down deeper down into your pelvis.

The pattern of contractions varies. One scenario is that at the beginning of labour they may only happen every 35-40 minutes or so and last just 10 seconds, then at the end, just before you give birth, they may come every minute or two and last 60 seconds. Alternatively, you may find that your labour begins with mild contractions about three minutes apart, and as your labour moves along they still have the same short gap in between them, but are gradually growing more powerful.

Staying comfortable early on

Just how much early contractions hurt depends on different things, many under your control but some not. The following can all make a major difference:
■ How relaxed and calm you are.
■ How physically comfortable you are.
■ What position you are sitting, standing or lying in.
■ Whether you are in your own home or have gone into hospital.
■ Whether you have some privacy and peace.

21

- If you have someone you like and trust with you.
- Whether you are using any pain-relieving/coping techniques of your own.
- Whether you are using any pain-relieving drugs yet.

It also depends on whether your contractions started naturally and gradually, or whether they are being helped along with medication (doctors call this artificial augmentation, or artificial acceleration of labour). Natural contractions tend to hurt less than those that are started or strengthened with drugs.

Early labour

People often wonder when they should call their midwife or go to hospital once their labour has begun. If in doubt, telephone for advice (the maternity ward if you are planning to have your baby in hospital, or your community/independent midwife if you are planning a home birth). If you are going into hospital, as a general guide it is usually best to wait until your contractions are about 15-20 minutes apart.

If you have had a baby before, you will probably give birth to your next babies faster. If you are going into hospital, set off when your contractions are coming every 20-25 minutes to be sure of getting there in time to make the best use of the facilities, including certain types of pain relief.

For first labours, and some subsequent ones, it can take several hours before contractions are regular enough to even call the hospital, and you certainly don't need to go in as soon as they start unless you would especially like to. In very early labour many women find they are happy just to carry on with ordinary gentle activities such as going for a walk, cooking, tidying up, playing with any children they have already, or just having a long, relaxing warm bath or shower.

Some women also find they want to start cleaning vigorously. The stories of mothers in labour feeling a strong desire to scrub kitchen floors are true, and it's thought to be part of a powerful natural instinct to get the nest in order before the baby comes.

Get set, go!
When your contractions become regular and much closer together, or the pain begins in the small of your back and radiates right around to the front just above your pubic bone, it is time to contact your hospital or midwife.

Many mothers have said that it was difficult to know what to do with themselves in very early labour (medical staff call it the 'latent' phase, and tell you your labour is not yet 'established'). It was too early to call a midwife or get in the car, but their contractions were beginning to come, so many activities were no longer an option. Luckily, there are plenty of things you can do to help you relax and ease any discomfort or pain you may be feeling. These things also help pass the time, which is more useful than it first sounds, because this latent phase can last for many hours, sometimes for as long as a day or two. And all that waiting can become tiring after a while, not to mention pretty boring.

Taking your mind off it – what helps

Distraction therapy (DT) can be especially useful now. There are several different sorts, ranging from simply watching a good film on video to visualisation exercises. DT works by helping you focus your mind on something other than the discomfort or pain you are in. Although it is simple, it can be highly effective, which is why it is one of the main techniques used in powerful self-help techniques such as self-hypnosis, meditation and autogenic training (p117)

People use DT to help themselves handle a wide variety of otherwise stressful or painful situations. For instance, researchers have found that playing videos to adult patients having painful dressings changed helps them cope better, and children on hospital paediatric units are far less conscious of the pain they are in when they are absorbed in a video game.

The pain is real enough, and it is still there, but the distraction ensures the person does not register so much of it. By giving the brain other interesting things (sounds, visual images) to deal with, it registers fewer of the pain signals, which means the person feels less pain.

Dentists have been using DT for many years, too. Many now play soothing music or show MTV to patients who are having work done on their teeth, and generally these

Distraction therapies at home
TV or videos; favourite relaxing music; video games; massage; visualisation; breathing exercises; relaxation techniques; self-hypnosis; and fairly easy board or card games. Scrabble is a classic DT for labour, as it manages to be both calming and absorbing.

patients need fewer pain-killing injections and appear calmer than those who are not offered DT. For the same reason some maternity units have now installed videos and TVs in their labour rooms, not just in the unit's sitting room.

If you have learned relaxation or visualisation techniques, autogenic training, breathing-for-labour methods or self-hypnosis, now is an excellent time to use these skills. Ask someone close to you to give you a shoulder and neck massage, pointing out any useful reflexology or shiatsu points to press in early labour if you know where they are. If you have any relaxing aromatherapy oils that are suitable for labour, such as Lavender, use them in the massage. Or add them to a warm bath (not hot as this could raise your baby's temperature).

All of these things will help you stay as relaxed and loose as possible between contractions. If you have a TENS machine it's a good idea to begin using it now to encourage the build-up of your body's own natural painkillers, endorphins.

The First Stage of Your Labour

The first stage of your labour is when your body creates the birth canal – a smooth, open passageway made from your womb, your dilated (open) cervix and your vagina. In the second stage of labour your womb's contractions push your baby down this birth canal and out into the world to be born.

Your cervix, the muscular gateway at the bottom, or neck, of your womb, has been doing a remarkable job over the last nine months, staying closed to hold in the increasing weight of your baby and the sac of amniotic fluid that surrounds her inside your body. Yet in just the few hours of labour it transforms itself from your baby's guardian into an open birth tunnel. It has to make this change fast by stretching from closed, or almost closed, to 10cm wide. This is one of the reasons why contractions in labour hurt, while the practice ones you get during pregnancy don't.

In most women the cervix stays closed until they go into labour. However, because of the increasing pressure of the growing baby's weight pressing down on it from above,

No pain
According to research by Russian obstetrician Velvoski, up to 10% of Russian mothers say that during labour they are only conscious of major physical effort and 'something happening' – not pain as such.

some women may have already dilated as much as 2cm before labour begins. Yet it can take others, especially first-time mothers, several long hours to get to that point. If a woman's cervix begins to open even more than this too early in pregnancy, her obstetrician may put a small dissolving surgical stitch there to help prevent her from going into premature labour.

Your amazing womb

To understand how your womb makes your cervix open up, imagine taking a stocking with a small hole in the toe, pulling it up over your foot, then continuing to pull gently and intermittently. Your big toe would make the hole in the stocking slightly bigger each time you pulled it.

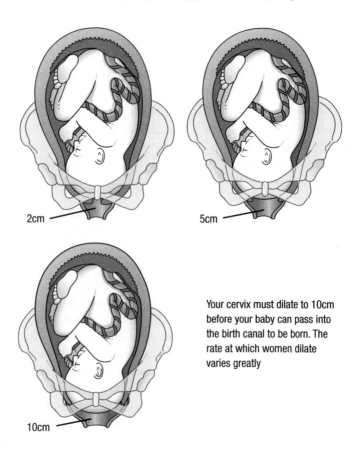

2cm

5cm

10cm

Your cervix must dilate to 10cm before your baby can pass into the birth canal to be born. The rate at which women dilate varies greatly

And as you went on doing so, that hole would become big enough for your other toes, and eventually your entire foot, to pass through. Something similar happens to your cervix when you are in labour, except that it closes up again neatly within a few short hours after your baby has been born.

Each time your womb contracts it pulls on your cervix, helping it to dilate, but this does not always happen evenly. A cervix can go from tightly shut to wide open in fits and starts because, just like with the rest of childbirth, dilation is a highly individual process that varies from woman to woman. One mother may go very slowly from 2cm to 5cm, then progress very fast to 10cm, while another may go quickly to 5cm then stop there for a while before moving on.

If you are having a second or subsequent baby, you may find that your cervix dilates very fast, especially after you have reached the 5cm mark.

How much does it really hurt?

When asked how much their labour pain hurts, women's replies range from 'excruciating' and 'no-one told me it would be like this', to 'not half as bad as I expected' and 'I can't understand why people make such a big thing of it'.

An important thing to know about labour pain is that it comes and goes. Unlike the pain caused by, say, slamming your hand in a door, which will hurt constantly, you are given opportunities to rest with labour pain (unless the process is being accelerated with drugs).

'They don't call it "labour" for nothing, but you find you can handle it'

At the beginning of your labour you will have rests of 15-20 minutes before your next contraction begins. Towards the end of the first stage, contractions will probably be coming every couple of minutes. Any pain will start gently and then gradually get stronger over the next 30-60 seconds, peak for perhaps 10 seconds, then start to die away, finally stopping altogether. Then you can rest for a while.

As labour progresses your contractions will become strong enough to make you stop moving and want to bend over, lean against something, practise relaxation breathing,

That familiar feeling
Even first-baby labour pain may feel reassuringly familiar. Many women say the pains in the first stage are like period pains, only stronger.

squat down or get down on all fours until the feeling passes. Some women also get very tired and prefer to lie down for a rest in between contractions, ideally on their left side to encourage the maximum blood supply to reach their baby. You will probably find you cannot continue talking through these later contractions, and that they will take your breath away.

Because labour pains are gradual, wave-like and intermittent, you will have time to prepare yourself to cope as you feel one beginning, whether by practising breathing or relaxation techniques, requesting extra back rubbing, or reaching out for the gas and air.

It helps to know that, at its most intense, the pain will not last long, perhaps just 10 seconds, after which it will gradually subside.

Transition

Towards the end of the first stage your womb changes the way it is working, from contractions that make it smaller and open up your cervix, to the powerful expulsive contractions that push your baby out to be born. Many obstetricians feel that this transitional stage is a separate, or fourth, major stage of labour in its own right. It can last for anything from a few minutes to one hour.

You may not notice it at all, but some mothers have strong emotions and sensations. Some feel sick or have diarrhoea. Others shake uncontrollably or feel cold. You may find your contractions don't seem to have a pattern to them anymore, that it no longer seems possible to cope with them, or that you suddenly feel confused, irritable and upset. Some women remember that they just wanted to go home, and found it difficult to co-operate with those around them, or even hear what was being said to them. You may find, too, that you don't want to be touched, helped or comforted, but just want to be left alone. Or you may feel re-energised as you see the end of your labour approaching. You might also notice an urge to push – though it is too soon to do so yet – possibly because your baby's head is now pressing hard on your rectum.

Nearly there

At this point your baby's head will be right down in the cavity within your pelvis. Occasionally, a small area of cervix has still not dilated out of the way, or has done so unevenly and left a small area behind. This is called a lip. If you get an urge to push your baby out when this lip is in place, it will become swollen, making it difficult to finish dilating.

To help stop yourself from pushing at this point, try getting on all fours with your head touching the ground and your bottom in the air. Breathing gas and air (p75) may give some pain relief and also stop the urge to push.

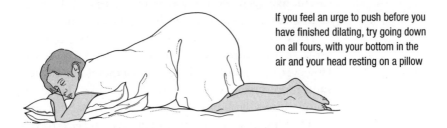

If you feel an urge to push before you have finished dilating, try going down on all fours, with your bottom in the air and your head resting on a pillow

What being in labour really feels like

In 1994 mothers at St George's Hospital, London, were asked to describe what it felt like to have a baby. Here are some of their comments on the first stage: 'not painful – I just felt like my stomach was heaving'; 'a dull ache in my lower back'; 'slicing, sideswiping pains'; 'a grinding, sickening, heavy ache in my back and belly'; 'slicing pain across the top of my pubic hair area'; 'stabs of sharp pain going down my inside thighs'; 'like a fat cord being pulled increasingly tighter, then releasing around my middle'; 'I just thought it was bad wind'.

Eating and drinking

In the past many hospitals would not let women eat anything when they were in labour. Because childbirth is usually such a huge physical effort, this sometimes meant that women who were in labour for a long time would become hungry and short of the calories they needed to

Thirsty work

Hospitals are usually very warm with dry air so you and your partner may get quite thirsty. It's a good idea to have a big bottle of cool, still spring water with you so you can take regular sips.

fuel the task they were undertaking. They would then become exhausted, perhaps too much so to continue their labours without medical intervention. The result was not infrequently a Caesarean section or instrumental, or assisted, delivery to pull their baby out (with forceps, for example).

The original rationale behind the old 'no eating' principle was a safety issue, based on the slight possibility that if an emergency Caesarean under general anaesthetic was necessary, the woman might vomit. When someone under general anaesthetic is sick there is a risk of inhaling the stomach's contents into the lungs, which would flood with fluid as a result. However, this can usually be avoided by careful management of the tube that is passed down an anaesthetised patient's throat during the operation.

These days most midwives and obstetricians have no problem with women in early labour having a light snack. However, once labour really gets going they advise against solid food, but may suggest isotonic drinks. These are energy drinks developed for sports players. Because they tend to contain a good balance of glucose and electrolytes they provide valuable energy without dehydrating you, which other sweet drinks, such as colas and sweet tea, can do. If you would like to have one to hand when you are in labour, perhaps try a few in the last part of your pregnancy to see which ones you like best.

Most women are too busy in labour to think about eating. However, you may find you'd like something light to eat at intervals. Some American Indian midwives offer warm soups, a Lepcha mother would be offered a high-protein snack such as meat from a fowl or goat, and if a Vietnamese mother is tiring she would be offered a bowl of rice with an egg. Good foods for British women include those high in complex carbohydrates, as they release their energy slowly and steadily into the system. Try a banana, a few digestive biscuits, chicken soup or wholemeal sandwiches of honey, peanut butter or any other favourite filling.

It's important to always let your midwife know if you have had something to eat.

The Second Stage of Your Labour

The second stage of your labour is when your baby is actually born, and starts after your cervix is fully dilated to 10cm. As you go into the second stage your contractions will probably feel about the same all the way through, instead of building up to a climax and tailing off. And you may feel an extra burst of energy and a strong, often irresistible urge to push, or 'bear down'.

If your baby is in the ideal position, the narrowest part of his head, which also measures about 10cm across, will lead as he is pushed slowly and steadily through your open cervix, as if through the polo neck of a jumper, and down your birth canal.

Your birth canal is not a straight tube but a curved one rather like the U-bend in a drainpipe. Nor is it equally wide all the way along. At the top it is widest from side to side, but at the outlet (the exit of the vagina) it is widest from front to back. This means that your baby's head and shoulders have to rotate and turn as he comes down. This happens naturally as your baby moves along, following

How long?
From being fully dilated to giving birth can take just a matter of minutes or as long as three hours. For most women it usually takes between half an hour to an hour.

Long labours

One in 10 labours is recorded as 'long' in the UK, but the definition of this varies depending on which hospital you are in and which consultant is looking after you.

the muscle and bony walls of your pelvis, but it can take a little while.

How your baby moves down the birth canal

If positioned in your womb with his head down and his back facing outwards, as most babies are, your baby's journey down the birth canal is likely to be as follows:

At first your baby's head is flexed, with his chin resting against his chest. This means the narrowest part of his head (about 10cm) is leading the rest of his body down into your pelvis. If, however, his head is not well flexed, the leading part will measure nearer 13cm across, which can make things more difficult

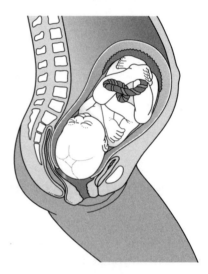

As your baby's head reaches your pelvic floor it turns by about 90° to face the base of your spine. His head then passes under your pubic bone and into the top of your vagina. It then extends upwards, like a diver coming up for air in slow motion, and after coming down a little further appears in the outside world

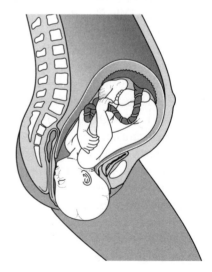

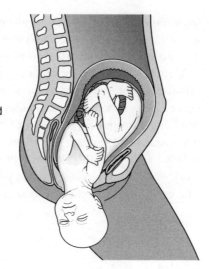

Your baby rotates sideways as his shoulders enter your pelvis. They need to follow the same turning motion as his head did. This usually happens quite quickly, with the midwife holding his head gently but firmly to support it. Your baby now turns and faces your thigh, as his shoulders are delivered. The rest of his body follows smoothly and easily

How you may be feeling

Do not worry if you are not able to co-ordinate your push-ing very well – your womb will still be doing most of the work automatically. Many women who have had an epidural and have little or no sensation in their lower body still manage to deliver their babies without extra help.

During the second stage you might feel as though you want to open your bowels. This is caused by the strong pressure of your baby's head against your rectum, which is usually empty anyway as faeces tend to be stored a few inches further up in the colon. However, there is no need to worry if you do move your bowels slightly – this is quite common and it is not going to be a surprise to your midwife or doctor. They will take little notice of it, and just whisk any faecal matter swiftly away with a piece of gauze.

Assisted delivery

Your baby may need some extra help in making his final entry into the world. If so, your obstetrician or midwife may suggest an assisted delivery, in which a medical instru-ment is used to help pull the baby out.

There are several reasons why this may need to be done, but two of the most common are that your baby is becoming short of oxygen and needs to be delivered quickly, or that you have had an overly long labour and are becoming too exhausted to push hard enough.

Ventouse (vacuum extraction) delivery is used most often, in about seven out of 10 cases where extra help is needed. This involves placing a suction cap on the baby's head. In a forceps delivery a pair of large, shallow spoons, like metal salad servers, are placed on either side of the baby's head. In both cases, the doctor or midwife will work with your pushes, easing your baby out gently. Currently, one in 10 mothers has an assisted delivery.

Ventouse delivery
It can take several minutes to apply the suction cap of a ventouse to a baby's head. Once attached, however, it can take just a couple of pushes to deliver the baby

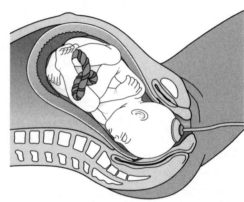

Forceps delivery
There are different types of forceps for different situations, but all encourage the baby to move down the birth canal and out into the world

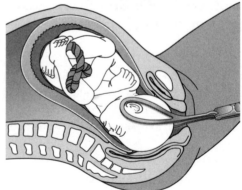

Your baby's first breath

When your baby first comes into contact with air the change in temperature makes him automatically take a breath and fill his lungs. It may take a little time before he is breathing efficiently and easily. If your baby's breathing is being affected by mucus in his nose or throat, the staff will check and clear this. If he needs any extra help your hospital will have all the necessary resuscitation equipment, plus the antidotes for any problems caused by pain-relieving drugs such as pethidine, which can sometimes interfere with a baby's breathing and suckling for a few days.

How can something that size come out of something this size?

Many women worry about this at some point during their pregnancy. While they know that this is what happens and that it is what has happened for many thousands of years for several billion women, the idea of something the size of a baby's head passing down a slim passageway like a vagina seems somehow beyond all reason. But your body is ingenious and adaptable. It has been designed to make such a thing possible because:

■ Your pelvic tissues have by now become very elastic, thanks to the influence of the 'relaxing hormone' progesterone throughout your pregnancy.

■ The pelvic tissues usually have all the time they need to stretch slowly and gently.

■ There are several different birth positions that can encourage your pelvis to open up naturally as wide as possible. These include variations on squatting upright, which your partner and midwife can help you to do when the time comes.

Your vagina, too, can stretch well. As your baby is coming down, your vagina's surface, which is made up of many folds of soft elastic tissue, stretches steadily apart and the tissues of your perineum (the area of skin and muscle between your vagina and anus) fan out. This means your baby will pass down a little of the way at each contraction, but slide back part of the distance he has come when the contraction stops.

Boosting
Women can sometimes start feeling tired out and discouraged during the second stage, and it is now that you may need all the encouragement and praise that your partner and midwife can give.

'The right words at the right time can keep you going when you think you're too tired to carry on. And my midwife knew just what I needed to hear'

Time of arrival

The favourite time to arrive for most babies is about 2am.

It can be frustrating and disheartening to watch or feel your baby's head coming down only to have it disappear back up again. But there is a good reason for this 'two steps forward, one step back' progress. It gives your pelvic tissues the chance to stretch gradually to accommodate your baby moving down, and so reduces the risk of tearing.

Preventing perineal tears and performing episiotomies

About one in three women does not experience even the smallest tear during labour. And where minor tears do occur, the blood supply to the perineum is so good that they usually heal within a couple of weeks without needing stitches. Larger tears are usually repaired with dissolving stitches.

One measure doctors take to reduce the risk of a bad tear is to perform an episiotomy. This is a surgical cut made through the perineum from the vagina, and about one in seven women has one during labour in the UK. An episiotomy may also be carried out to speed up the second stage as it creates more room for the baby's head to emerge. And if a woman has an assisted delivery, it may be done to make a little extra room to slide in the ventouse or forceps. You do not feel the cut either because the area is anaesthetised or because the stretching in the region is so intense that you do not feel the pain signals.

However, the cut needs stitching afterwards and some women have reported that if the area is not properly

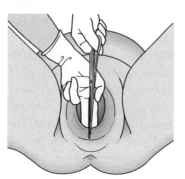

An episiotomy is done as the baby's head appears. The cut is usually made either straight down, towards the anus, or angled to the left or right of the anus

anaesthetised this can hurt even more than the labour itself. Further, the stitched perineum is likely to feel sore while it is healing, and it can take from two to eight weeks, sometimes longer, before the area is comfortable again. So it is something most mothers prefer to avoid. A debate continues to rage about whether many episiotomies are being performed unnecessarily.

Fortunately, there are several things you can do in the weeks leading up to your labour that may help reduce the risk of tearing, over-stretching or having an episiotomy:

■ Do as many pelvic floor exercises as you can throughout your pregnancy. Your pelvic floor is the sling of muscles that holds up your abdominal organs and the growing weight of your baby. Exercises that target this area are invaluable in strengthening it for childbirth and also for encouraging a quick recovery. An added bonus is that they help prevent the incontinence problems that one in three mothers develops, both as a result of pregnancy and because the huge physical effort of pushing their baby out has weakened their pelvic floor.

■ Massage oil into your perineal area. This should be done every day for about six weeks or so before the birth. Cold-pressed olive oil and wheat germ oil, available from large supermarkets and health shops, are both good choices as they are rich and thick. If you can't massage yourself, possibly because your bump is too large to comfortably reach beneath it, ask your partner to do it.

With a few drops of oil on your fingers and thumb, slide your thumb gently inside your vagina against its back wall. With your forefinger on the perineum (the area between your vagina and anus) massage gently, trying to stretch your vaginal opening. Spend about five minutes each day doing this. As time goes on, try increasing the number of fingers you place inside your vagina as this will help to stretch the skin even more.

■ Make a birthplan. This is a written record of how you

Your baby's size

Most babies only grow to the size of their environment, so a small, slim mother is likely to have a smaller baby (unless she is diabetic). Nearly all singleton babies weigh between 5 ½lbs and 10lbs, with the average being 7-8lbs. Only one in 20 weighs 10lbs or more.

would like your birth to be handled, provided no unforeseen medical issues come up while you are in labour that mean a change of plan. Your birthplan stays in your folder of maternity notes for the midwife who will be with you during your labour to look at. It's usually set out as a series of numbered points that explain your wishes regarding all the different aspects of your labour, and it needs to be signed by both you and the obstetrician who is overseeing your pregnancy. Points might include:

'I made a birthplan but was too busy in labour to think about it. My partner kept checking it, though, to make sure everything was as I'd hoped it would be'

- The pain relief you would like to use.
- Whether you would like to move about freely.
- The position you would like to give birth in.
- Whether you are happy to have your labour accelerated with drugs or would prefer to avoid this unless it was absolutely medically necessary.
- Whether you would mind any trainee midwives or doctors watching you, or caring for you, in labour.
- The names of anyone you would like with you.
- Whether you want to avoid having an episiotomy unless it was medically unavoidable, and would rather experience small tears in your perineum and labial areas instead.
- Whether you would like to use a complementary therapy.

- Check your hospital's record on episiotomies. Some carry out far more than others. If you are planning a hospital birth check its episiotomy rates by asking the consultant you are booked with, your local Community Health Council, whose job it is to monitor all aspects of hospital practice in your area, or the Director of Midwifery Services at the hospital. You could also ask a junior member of the consultant's team or your midwife, perhaps while having an antenatal check-up with them.

Some consultant obstetricians, and the team of doctors under them, are also more likely to carry out episiotomies than others. The reason is often, but not always, because they practise at hospitals that deliver a larger amount of babies using forceps or ventouse, which usually require an episiotomy.

■ Try birthing positions that are variants of squatting. The least helpful position to have your baby in is lying on your back. Getting into an upright or semi-upright squatting (not sitting) position, supported by your midwife and partner, may help to deliver your baby in a controlled and gentle way that will be less likely to cause a tear or make an episiotomy necessary.

Check out your local yoga and natural birthing groups (usually run by The National Childbirth Trust and the Active Birth movement) for help and practical advice on squatting positions in labour. Discuss it with your midwife in an antenatal appointment. You may find it comfortable to squat supported by your partner and/or midwife, perhaps placing a cushion under each heel for support. Ask if your hospital has a birth cushion – this is a wedge-shaped piece of foam, with a 'V' removed from the middle, held in a light tubular steel frame with padded arms. Designed by UK obstetrician Jason Gardosi, a birth cushion can be a godsend as it helps you sit in a squatting position without straining your leg muscles.

■ Support your perineum. Ask your midwife to apply gentle but firm counter-pressure to your perineum as your baby's head crowns. Crowning comes towards the

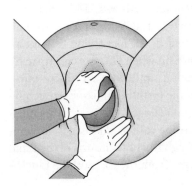

Ask your midwife to apply counter-pressure to your perineum as your baby emerges to reduce the likelihood of tears

Home births and episiotomies

It's thought that fewer episiotomies are carried out during home births because mothers are more relaxed and better able to move around freely and adopt birth-friendly positions. These usually create more room for the baby's head to come down.

end of labour, when your baby's head is pushing its way past the perineum and appears as a widening domed circle in your vagina. Pushing gently back against this helps restrain the baby's head from being pushed out too suddenly. If it emerges more slowly, the perineal tissues are given more time to stretch.

■ Have your baby at home, provided there is no good medical reason why you need to be in hospital. A 1998 study of 1068 first- and second-time mothers in New York who had home births found that seven out of 10 didn't have any perineal tears and only 1.4% needed an episiotomy (the average US figure is 50%).

■ Give birth in water. Natural birth pioneer Janet Balaskas believes that giving birth in warm water results in fewer tears and reduces the need for an episiotomy. This may be because the warmth of the water softens the perineal tissues and encourages them to stretch more easily.

■ For the same reason, ask your midwife or partner to hold comfortingly hot compresses against your perineal area during the second stage.

■ Try visualisation exercises (p128), seeing your perineum and vagina in your mind's eye as soft and stretching easily.

What giving birth really feels like

The sensations you feel in the second stage of your labour come from the powerful pushing you are doing and from the stretching of your vagina, perineum and labia. The women in a survey carried out at St George's Hospital, London, in 1994 described it as: 'like trying to pass an enormous, hard bowel motion when I'm very constipated'; 'like trying to pass a melon out'; 'like a Chinese burn' (describing the feeling of the birth canal tissues stretching wide); 'a splitting, tearing feeling'; 'a massive stretching, but no pain' (this is often the case as the tissues are temporarily stretched far enough to obliterate any of the usual neurological pain messages from them); 'nothing much – I had an epidural'.

The Third Stage of Your Labour

The third stage of your labour begins after your baby has been born, and is when you deliver your placenta. As more strong contractions shrink your womb even further, your placenta crumples up and peels away from the wall of the womb, rather like a large sticky label peeling away from a deflating balloon.

Your midwife may hasten this process along by giving you an injection of artificial oxytocin (oxytocin is one of the hormones that makes your womb contract) to stimulate strong contractions. But it will usually happen naturally within an hour or so of giving birth if your doctor and midwife can be persuaded to be patient.

As the placenta comes away, the blood vessels that have been supplying it throughout your pregnancy will become exposed, leading to some blood loss. However, they will close down rapidly as your womb continues to shrink.

Your midwife may also pull on the umbilical cord to which your placenta is still attached to encourage it to come away. She does this very gently so as not to cause a haemorrhage. The placenta is then delivered through your vagina.

Back to normal
It takes a few weeks for your womb to get back to its usual shape and size. By then it will have shrunk from the size and shape of a very large melon to nearer that of a fig.

Finishing touches

If you have had an episiotomy or suffered any tears, these will be treated once your placenta has been delivered. According to the National Birthday Trust's major survey on pain relief in labour in 1990, the sewing-up of tears after birth can hurt almost as much as labour itself. However, if the area is properly anaesthetised you shouldn't feel a thing. It is vital that anaesthetic is given enough time to work – from three to six minutes on average. If you can feel any pain after this time, insist on more anaesthetic.

Pain – Why Have Any?

These days there are many different ways to help you have a smooth and comfortable labour. This book looks at 25 of them, and there are probably even more than this. Yet it seems like a fundamental design fault in human physiology that having a baby hurts in the first place. Christian religion used to try to explain it away by saying it was a punishment bestowed on all the daughters of Eve for leading Adam astray.

This may sound ridiculous now, but as little as 300 years ago midwives who made herbal medicines to ease labour pain – and the mothers who took them – could be prosecuted and punished. The punishments were sometimes very severe indeed.

One such case involved a mother in Scotland who was having a difficult labour with twins. After the birth, on the orders of the local Church Elders, she was burned at the stake for taking pain-relieving herbs. Her crime, so they wrote in their record books, was 'cheating Heaven of the cries of the righteous which rise up to Him in times of

Help at hand
Labour usually hurts, and it does so for solid physical and psychological reasons. But there is plenty that can be done to make it a lot more comfortable and even obliterate the pain – by doctors, midwives, complementary therapies and, perhaps most of all, by you yourself.

43

trouble, and which are His due'. In other words, it was felt that the distress of women in childbirth was natural and belonged to God, and to deprive Him of His dues in this area was an act of severe heresy.

The Establishment still seemed to feel the same way just 150 years ago, too, as the surgeon who introduced chloroform to women in labour was roundly criticised by many of the elders of the Church of England. Even today, mothers who choose to have an epidural right away may still occasionally come across someone who clearly feels this is somehow a bit decadent.

Why labour hurts at all

Labour can hurt because of the following:

■ Contractions themselves. As your womb muscles contract they irritate the nerve fibres that are threaded through them.

■ The position your baby is in. There are good ones and not so good ones. Most babies are in the classic head-down position, with their back facing outwards towards the world when labour starts. If the baby is in a different position, perhaps breech (bottom-first), labour can be more difficult and potentially more painful.

■ Your cervix is flattening out (effacing) and stretching open (dilating).

■ Your pelvic tissues are all stretching – ligaments, soft tissues and joints – which upsets the nerves running through them.

■ Your muscles are becoming short of oxygen. There is not enough oxygen-rich blood flowing in and out of your womb muscles when they are working hard in labour. Normally, arterial blood coming directly from your heart and lungs brings vital oxygen to the womb muscles, and also food which they convert to energy. The deoxygenated blood flows out of muscles afterwards, taking any cell waste products with it. But this flow is interrupted in labour because when the muscles of the womb contract powerfully they squeeze the blood vessels running through them, partially cutting off both the oxygenated blood flowing *in* and the deoxygenated blood flowing *out*. This area of muscle then becomes ischaemic (oxygen-starved) and goes into spasm, which hurts.

■ When your womb muscles contract, the metabolic rate of all the tissues in the surrounding area increases, which in turn speeds up the onset of pain.

■ Tension. This builds up in your muscles during labour, making them sore. Many women automatically stiffen and hunch their shoulders at the peak of a major contraction, developing painful shoulders and an aching back as a result. When muscles become stiff or tired they are more vulnerable to injury such as tears and strains. Regular massage of the neck, shoulders and back can help, as can good support for the back and being in a comfortable position.

■ The pushing apart of the pelvic joints as your baby comes down the birth canal, and the stretching of tissues in your vagina, vulva and perineum as your baby is being born can cause pain. However, many women say that during their second stage of labour, especially towards the end of it, they were not aware of pain as such, but more of the effort of pushing. It may hurt more if your baby has a particularly large head, if she is a very big baby (which can happen when the mother is diabetic), or if you have a particularly small pelvic cavity.

Why labour hurts some women less than others

This has nothing whatsoever to do with bravery. There are many different factors that can, and do, affect the amount of pain you feel:

■ Whether you have had a baby before. In second or subsequent births your cervix will open up more easily, your vagina and perineum will stretch a little more readily, and your labour should be much quicker and easier than your first.

Some mothers say that their body seems to remember what to do second time around, and it is certainly true

Pain tolerance
People don't have different pain thresholds (a fixed level at which they feel pain). What they do have is a higher or lower pain tolerance, and many different things can influence that.

that you are less likely to have problems with the birth getting started properly or with contractions that are not being very effective. And because you will understand childbirth better, you will probably be a lot more relaxed and confident than you were first time around.

■ How old you are. Research shows that giving birth can be less painful for younger women.

'I didn't believe what my friends kept telling me, that the second one is much easier. But it's true'

■ What your periods are like. If you tend to have mild periods, you may be more likely to have an easier time in labour.

■ How much you understand about what is happening to you. Women know far more about childbirth now than they did 30 years ago, thanks to more antenatal/parentcraft classes, the work of The National Childbirth Trust and Active Birth organisations, and the huge number of books and magazines about pregnancy, birth and babies. Mothers now usually understand far more about what is happening to their body during labour and can work *with* it rather than against it. This is partly why labour has become much shorter since the early 1960s.

■ How confident you are feeling in your ability to manage labour.

■ How much you are able to consciously relax and stay calm.

■ What your mother and friends say about their own labours, if they discuss them at all.

Shorter labours

Labours are getting quicker. Over the last 40 years the average time for first labours has dropped from 10 hours to seven, and for subsequent labours from nine hours to four.

Towards the end of their pregnancy, many women report feeling remarkably calm and unworried about childbirth. Many describe the feeling as like being cocooned against the rest of the world. This is thought to be the mind and body's way of helping pregnant women feel relaxed and confident. Otherwise, just the expectation of pain or problems can make a perfectly normal labour hurt more. Hearing positive stories about friends' and relatives' childbirths can all add to your natural instinctive confidence that you will be able to manage just fine. But other people's 'what I went through' accounts (which many seem eager to share with you as soon as you mention you're pregnant) generally have the opposite effect.

If people insist on telling you their experiences in detail and you don't much want to hear them, either ask them to pick a more helpful subject or try to think 'they're talking about themselves, not me. Their lives aren't exactly like mine, their personalities and circumstances aren't. So why should our childbirths be the same?'

The memory of a previous childbirth that did not go very well can also knock your confidence. Try to think 'that was then, this is now', and know that second births usually go far more smoothly and feel a good deal easier.

> ' "I was on that delivery table for 27 hours and had all these stitches. The nurses said he was really big – 11lbs – for someone my size. You look like you're having a big one, too," said my mother-in-law the week before I went into labour. She scared the living daylights out of me. Yet when I finally had Ben he was all of 6lbs 13oz and took just 10 hours'

- Your culture. When Liverpool Maternity Hospital compared Nordic and Slav women's experiences of childbirth with the way Italian women felt, it found a vast difference. In Italy it is widely accepted that a labouring woman can make as much noise as she needs to as a way of coping. But women from Nordic countries seem to approach labour in a far more controlled way, often saying little even when they are in great pain.
- Whether you have been given any drug treatment, such as an artificial oxytocin drip, to make your contractions stronger and speed up your childbirth.

Contractions induced by a drip tend to hurt more than natural ones. They will be strong right from the beginning, and come close together straightaway, instead of beginning more mildly with long gaps in between then gradually becoming stronger and closer together. And there is no gradual build-up to their peak intensity – they will be full-on almost immediately.

The remarkable power of relaxation

If a woman is reasonably calm and relaxed during her childbirth, any labour pains she feels can be dramatically reduced. Yet if she becomes distressed or frightened, the amount of tension in her muscles increases and the level of natural pain-killing opiates (endorphins) produced by her nervous system drops, making her labour more painful and more distressing.

When that happens her body begins to produce a different group of hormones. These are substances called catecholamines and they include adrenaline. They would normally be released in the second stage of labour to stimulate the powerful, expulsive contractions of the womb that push the baby out. If these hormones are made too early in the first stage they can inhibit the vital contractions that make the womb smaller and pull up and open out the cervix. This usually makes labour longer and so more exhausting, which also tends to make it hurt more.

Catecholamines also cause another problem. Because they are pain transmitters, too, the more of them you produce, the more pain you feel. And so pain's vicious circle continues:

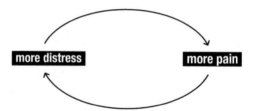

However, it is possible to break this cycle and set a positive one in motion instead:

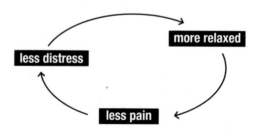

Drug-based pain relief can do this, since if you feel less pain you'll be less upset, more able to relax and better able to start producing more endorphins. Complementary therapies, such as homeopathy, that work gently on the emotions in labour may also break the cycle.

Further, what your mind can do, it can also undo. Effective self-help techniques that encourage relaxation, such as breathing techniques, visualisation, self-hypnosis and autogenic training, will help your body increase its endorphin production and reduce its catecholamine output.

Pain-killing drugs and you

As with other sorts of pain and medication, some of the drugs for soothing labour pain work better on some women than on others, and every mother's reaction to them is slightly different. So if you have already been given a standard shot of pain-relieving medication but you are still in pain, ask for more. Take no notice if you're told: 'Don't be silly, it can't possibly still be hurting'. Keep complaining. Or better still, sort out with your partner beforehand what he will do on your behalf should this happen. If his insistence doesn't get anywhere, he should ask to see the anaesthetist.

What your baby feels when she's being born

When a mother is in labour, everyone's attention is focused on what *she* is feeling. But what about the baby being squeezed by the contractions of what has been her peaceful home for 40 weeks, and then propelled down a birth canal? How does *she* feel?

It's difficult to know for sure. Many specialists are making educated guesses based on research studies of unborn babies and their mothers, and much of their thinking is documented in respectable specialist magazines such as *The Journal of Pre and Perinatal Psychology*. Contributors include experts in fetal (unborn baby) medicine who take a scientific approach, rebirthing therapists who help people solve psychological problems through reliving birth, and pre- and perinatal psychologists who are interested in the behaviour

Mind power
When your mind is on your side, it's an astonishingly powerful and effective ally. Self-help techniques such as relaxation and visualisation, breathing for labour and self-hypnosis can all help make sure your mind works *for* you, not against you.

of babies in the womb and soon after they are born.

Despite their different backgrounds, they are beginning to come to the same conclusion – that babies do feel their birth, and it is probably uncomfortable.

A baby being squeezed and crushed at intervals while inside a powerfully contracting, muscular womb, and then propelled down the birth canal may well feel some pain, or at least discomfort. You know what it's like when a doctor puts a blood-pressure cuff on your arm to take a reading? Fetal specialists suggest that, to a baby being born, one of your contractions might feel like having such a cuff wrapped around her entire body, inflated to the max and squeezing powerfully for 30 seconds or so every three to four minutes.

According to Dr Lennart Righard, consultant pediatrician at the University of Lund and Malmo General Hospital in Sweden: 'The unborn baby, including its brain and nerve system, is well developed long before birth, as you can see from Caesarean birth of premature infants. And when you see a very newborn baby it is obvious that labour and delivery are overwhelming and exhausting events for them.'

There are two main theories about unborn babies and their sensitivity to pain:

- To register pain as pain you need to have felt it before and remember it. Although unborn babies react to pain stimuli by flinching away, because they have no memory they do not actually feel what we would call pain.
- Unborn babies may well feel pain just like toddlers, children and adults do. Most doctors now accept that newborns certainly do, and many would ask what the difference is between an unborn 40-week-old baby coming down the birth canal and a baby of exactly the same age who's just been born. Estimates vary as to when unborn babies may start feeling pain – some experts suggest at just 17 weeks, while others go for a more cautious 26 weeks (despite the evidence of neo-natal specialists looking after premature babies in intensive care units who are born at only 23 or 24 weeks' gestation).

The second theory represents relatively new thinking. Only 30 years ago newborns who needed an emergency cardiac operation would be given open-heart surgery without anaesthetic. This is now regarded as barbaric because paediatricians know from checks recording the level of stress hormones present in those babies' bloodstreams when they underwent the operation that they were indeed in great pain. Further proof of this, if it was needed, comes from the fact that the newborns who were given anaesthetic recovered far better than those who weren't, and were less likely to die during or soon after the operation.

If babies do feel pain while their mother is in labour, we have to find a way to ease this. But it is very difficult to give an unborn baby painkillers. If the drugs are given via the mother, she would have to be given such a high dose that it would knock her out and might even affect some of the baby's vital functions, such as breathing.

At the moment the only thing obstetricians can do to reduce any discomfort an unborn baby might feel is to spray anaesthetic on her head if she has to have a monitoring clip attached there or if a blood sample has to be taken from one of the small vessels on her head.

Some say it is sentimental to think that babies might suffer at all while being born. They also suggest that it's pointless to worry about this anyway since the babies don't remember a thing about it afterwards. Or do they?

What mothers remember about giving birth

Conventional wisdom says that, unlike with other sorts of pain, women tend to forget labour pain quickly and completely thanks to the high levels of oxytocin in their system during the birth and for two or three days afterwards. Oxytocin is the amnesia hormone as well as the one that helps make your womb contract in labour. You have very high levels of it in your bloodstream while in childbirth, and some oxytocin crosses the placenta to your baby. It is said to help mothers forget about their labour, and it may do the same for the baby, too.

Yet research on the subject does not prove this. In fact,

Unborn babies are aware

Over the past 20 years researchers from around the world, including North America, Guatemala, Italy and Australia, have published studies in the field of prenatal psychology (see References). These suggest that unborn babies are awake and conscious in the womb and, once born, can remember and react to songs, music, voices, stories and even poetry that they heard there.

some studies show that women tend to remember a great deal about their labour, and that there is little wrong with their accuracy (see References).

What may happen instead is that most women are so happy to finally have their baby in their arms that all the pain and hard work is seen to have been worthwhile, so it is not really something that seems important any longer, even though it may have been very difficult at the time. Yet this is not the same as forgetting all about it. What's more, as little as 10 years ago the most popular form of pain relief in labour in the UK was pethidine, which is well known for its potential memory-altering effects. Even now one third of women still use it, and this may help in perpetuating the myth that 'it's all right – you won't remember it afterwards'.

> 'How am I to describe such a beautiful yet painful event when all I see and feel now is the beautiful part? The pain I felt during labour is all but forgotten'
>
> A new mother quoted in *Easing Labour Pain*, Harvard Common Press, 1992

What your baby may remember about being born

It may be that babies, too, remember more about being born than anyone gives them credit for. Studies also suggest that under regressional hypnosis children and adults can recall the labours that led up to their births, the births themselves and how they felt about it all remarkably clearly.

One piece of research in particular is food for thought. An obstetrician working in San Francisco called Dr David Cheek carried out an investigation involving more than 500 people he had delivered when he was a young obstetrician in Chico, California. Having first checked that the children had never been told anything about their births by their mothers, he put each into light regressional hypnosis, then took them back to their time in the womb and through their own birth.

He found that these men and women were able to tell and even show him the exact way they were born – the turns of their own head and shoulders as they came down the birth canal, whether they were born head-down, bottom-first or delivered by Caesarean, or whether they were helped out by ventouse or forceps. Some of the details they remembered were very specific, such as becoming stuck at a certain place, or turning in a particular way during the first half of the second stage. Their accounts matched the records that had been stored in Dr Cheek's private work files for the previous two decades – records that they had never seen and to which they had no access.

Another smaller study by Dr David Chamberlain, a San Diego psychologist specialising in prenatal work and past President of the International Society for Pre and Perinatal Psychology, used light hypnosis to help mothers and their children (ranging from nine to 23 years old) recall what the labours and children's births had been like. Again, the accounts were surprisingly coherent and detailed – and they matched.

Many of his subjects spoke about the discomfort and pain they felt while in the contracting womb, coming down the birth canal and being born. They recalled being squeezed, pushed and squashed, and also spoke about discomfort and/or pain in the neck, head and shoulder area, especially if they were helped out using steel forceps or ventouse suction equipment. One little boy, whose mother had a difficult birth, said it had left him 'exhausted, aching and stiff'. Another little girl said: 'It's dark... I'm getting a rush of energy... I feel like I'm going to explode! I feel like everything is rushing to my head.'

Some psychologists are convinced that children not only feel their births fully and can remember them, but that some who had a difficult time will act them out as they grow up to try to erase the memory and feeling of it. Psychotherapist William Emerson, who is a world authority in this area and is currently practising in California, gives one particular example of a little girl called Rowan whose parents came to him because she used to repeatedly cram herself into the corner of her cot and crush her head painfully against its wooden bars. Rowan's medical history revealed that her birth had been very difficult, and that she had been stuck for four-and-a-half hours, wedged in the birth canal.

Help prevent your unborn baby feeling pain

Although studies and reports like the ones mentioned here are fascinating, thought-provoking, and make perfectly good sense to most mothers and also to many progressive midwives and doctors, they do not prove beyond all doubt that babies experience pain, or even discomfort, when their mothers are giving birth to them.

And even if they do, it's unlikely to be the same pain you feel in labour. Your baby's abdominal muscles are not contracting like yours are, and her internal dimensions are not being stretched as yours are. However, she *is* being squeezed, and may experience uncomfortable pressure on her head as she crowns. Being delivered by forceps or ventouse is probably pretty uncomfortable, too. According to Professor Nicholas, Head of Obstetrics at Queen Charlotte's Hospital in London, if a 7lbs baby becomes stuck and needs an assisted delivery, a force of about 40lbs would need to be exerted on her head and neck.

Medical science has not yet found a way to give babies pain-killing drugs for their own births, but fortunately there are many other ways we can try to help them, based on the idea that what helps a mother in labour is also likely to help her baby. Your midwife or obstetrician, your partner and you yourself can work together to make sure that you have as smooth, uncomplicated and swift a labour as possible by:

■ Doing anything and everything possible to help your labour go as smoothly as possible. Experiencing many hours of ineffective contractions and pushing may be difficult and upsetting for your baby as well for as you.
■ Making sure you have all the pain relief that you personally need – a pain-free or reasonably comfortable mother may mean a more comfortable baby. It is no coincidence that babies born to mothers who have had epidurals are often born in considerably better shape than babies born to mothers who did not have adequate

pain relief when they needed it.

■ Doing anything that helps you stay as calm and as relaxed as possible could also makes things easier on your baby. This could be simply having someone you trust with you all the time, or using complementary therapies such as aromatherapy, acupuncture, massage, homeopathy, reflexology, self-hypnosis and autogenic training, or natural DIY techniques such as warm baths, water pools, visualisation, deliberate relaxation exercises and breathing for labour. (If you would like to find out more about any of these, please see the next half of the book, when we look in detail at the different methods of pain relief for childbirth.)

Calmer mothers, comfier babies

A few old-fashioned doctors still think the idea of 'calm mother equals calm unborn baby' is just wishful thinking. Yet there has been a good deal of research carried out by psychologists and even a few forward-thinking obstetricians (see References) to suggest that because unborn babies are inhabiting the same body as their mother, they are aware of any strong emotions she has and can be affected by them.

It is suggested that this is because there is deep communication between a mother and her unborn baby on two levels. The first is on a deep psychological or psychic level. The second is on a physical (biochemical) one, because the stress hormones you produce, such as cortisol and adrenaline, cross the placenta. When they reach your baby's system in sufficient quantities, which they can do quite rapidly, they can have a similar effect on your unborn child as they do on yourself. According to a report in the *International Journal of Prenatal and Perinatal Psychology and Medicine*: 'Unborn babies themselves are quick to pick up on their mother's thoughts. Just one example is that babies are more active when their mothers are awaiting ultrasound for an amniocentesis test than when waiting for ordinary ultrasound.'

Dr Valman of Northwick Park Hospital in London

Calming your unborn baby
American research involving more than 1000 mothers in 1992 by San Francisco obstetrician Dr David Cheek found evidence of telepathy between mothers and their unborn babies. Prenatal psychologists suggest mothers could use this in labour to send their baby 'it's OK' messages and so reduce any anxiety the baby might be feeling.

How babies respond

Researchers at the University of South Wales in Sydney carried out an experiment in 1994 involving a group of pregnant women watching some upsetting scenes from a film to see what, if anything, the unborn babies noticed. After just 20 minutes the babies began kicking wildly and their heart rates shot up.

carried out a study, published in the *British Medical Journal*, which showed that when a pregnant woman becomes anxious or upset, her unborn baby increases its level of sharp kicks and squirming movements by up to 10 times. Another, rather unkind, experiment was done by Austrian obstetrician Dr Emil Reinhold. A number of pregnant women were placed in a relaxed position and monitored by a scanner. Dr Reinhold then told each woman that her baby was not moving (which could have meant that the baby was resting, that there was something wrong or even that the baby had died). In every case this alarmed the woman so much that within a matter of a few seconds her unborn baby was kicking furiously.

It is arguable that if anxiety heightens pain for the baby as it does for the mother, soothing that anxiety may be helpful in reducing the amount of discomfort a baby might feel during its own birth.

The positive side of pain

If birth can be uncomfortable or painful for babies as well as their mothers, it seems extraordinary that evolution has allowed things to turn out this way. But some obstetricians suggest that the stress hormones a baby releases when she is being born (possibly prompted by the clenching and contracting of the womb's muscles and birth canal), help to stimulate her lungs to work and complete their maturing. This could partly explain why babies born by Caesarean are more likely to have initial breathing problems because they miss out on the breath-stimulating squeezing of ordinary labour.

Your Choices for Pain Relief During Childbirth

A decision about what sort of pain relief you'd like when you have your baby is often the last thing on a busy pregnant woman's list of 'things to sort out'. Yet thinking back to the day they had their babies, many women say if they'd known then what they know now, it would have been the first. Luckily, there are at least 25 ways to deal with labour pain, including pharmacological (drug-based) methods, such as a special type of epidural that allows you to walk around smiling, and self-help methods, such as breathing and self-hypnosis. The following pages look at them all – their pros, cons and how effective they are.

Pharmacological Methods

No-one but you knows what your labour feels like. There are as many different experiences as there are mothers. Small wonder, then, that the type of pain relief you use is an individual matter based on personal choice, how you are feeling, what is safe to use and what is available.

Just a few years ago the 'natural is good, drugs are bad' school of thought regarding childbirth was gaining ground, but fortunately today the attitude is more one of 'have whatever suits you'. Giving birth is an enormous personal achievement, whether you go through labour without any form of pain relief at all or need the strongest drugs available right from the start.

> 'In childbirth I am no Wonder Woman. Give me my drugs!'
>
> Madonna

'Too posh to push'

So sure are some women in the UK about how they want their child to be born that they are following the trend set

Keep an open mind

When it comes to pain relief, try to keep an open mind. No matter how much thought you have given the matter beforehand, or how well informed you are, you cannot be sure how you are going to feel until you are actually in labour.

by women in the USA. Some are quite clear that they want a spinal or epidural as soon as possible in their labour, while others pay privately to have an elective Caesarean, which means they will not go through labour or have any contractions.

A survey of 125,000 births carried out in a three-month period by the Royal College of Obstetricians in 2001 found that 7% of British women asked for a Caesarean where there was 'no good medical reason' for them to have one. The media jumped on this, calling the mothers 'too posh to push', and implying that Caesareans had become the fashionable way to have a baby after a series of glamorous rock and film stars had plumped for the procedure.

But those reports were only half-truths. The media ignored the fact that nine out of 10 of the mothers who had asked for a Caesarean had done so because they believed it would be the safest way for their baby to be delivered, and not because they did not want to have an ordinary vaginal birth for reasons of their own. Believing a Caesarean was safer for their baby was more important to them than the fact that they themselves would be having a major abdominal operation (albeit a very safe and common one), which carries its own discomforts, problems and a recovery period of three to 12 months.

Ask for whatever you need, whenever you need it

Another British study in 1987 looked at the type of pain relief mothers planned on having, and the type they actually did have when the time came. A number of women whose babies were soon due were asked whether they were planning to have an epidural. Most said they weren't. Yet the number who eventually ended up doing so was four times as many as originally thought would.

'I started off just with TENS, and when I was 5cm dilated got into the water pool, which was a huge relief, and had some gas and air. It was enough'

Similarly, a UK survey of 106 first-time mothers found that before they went into labour seven out of 10 were planning to use methods that offered partial relief, such as TENS and gas and air, and only one in 10 wanted an epidural. Yet after going into labour, fewer than two in 10 used TENS or gas and air, and six out of 10 had an epidural.

These figures probably reflect the fact that first labours tend to be slower than subsequent labours and are more likely to require drugs to encourage them on, and so are more painful. They also suggest that it's a good idea to keep your options open – try to be flexible in your plans for pain relief and have some back-up strategies.

Changing needs
You can usually switch to a different form of pain relief during labour whenever you want to. You don't have to stay with the same one throughout.

Epidurals and spinals

Epidurals and spinals are the most powerful, effective, reliable forms of pain relief for labour, and so are known as the Rolls Royce of anaesthetics. Both involve having an injection deep into the base of your back, and work by blocking the pain signals that would normally travel from your contracting womb to your brain. However, there are some important differences between them. This section looks at the differences so that you can make an informed decision about which might be right for you.

'I used breathing and TENS for 11 hours but was still only 2cm dilated, exhausted and getting nowhere. The obstetrician gave me a drip to make my contractions more powerful and that really hurt, so I had an epidural for the rest of the time, which was brilliant. And because I didn't have all that pain wiping me out, I even had enough energy to push Jenna out myself without them needing to use forceps'

There are three main types, all of which must be given by an anaesthetist:
- Standard epidural. This takes about 15-30 minutes to work. Your legs will gradually go numb so you need to stay in bed.
- A spinal. This provides instant relief. Your legs will go numb immediately so, again, you must be in bed.
- Mobile/walking, or combined, epidural. This is a mixture of a standard epidural and a spinal. Because you retain some of the sensation in your legs it's

possible to walk around. A more recent development is the mobile spinal, which is a further refinement of the mobile epidural.

Standard epidural

The word epidural comes from the ancient Greek word *epi*, meaning 'around', and with a standard epidural anaesthetic drugs are injected into the space around (not inside) the sac of fluid surrounding your spine. This space contains fatty material, blood vessels and nerve roots.

About one in five British mothers has an epidural. In some major hospitals it is nearer two in five, and in the USA it's nearly four in five. Twice as many first-time mothers have epidurals, possibly because their labours tend to be longer and more painful, or because they're more likely to be induced (started off) or accelerated (speeded up) with medication, which can produce very strong contractions straightaway.

How you have it

Epidurals are always given by an anaesthetist. You will be asked to sit forward or lie on your side, and bend your back into a 'C' shape by either leaning over your knees or bringing them towards your chest. This will help open up your back, ready for the needle to be put in. The anaesthetist will first inject the area with some local anaesthetic to numb it. This may sting briefly but from then on you shouldn't feel any pain, only pressure as the epidural needle slides in. An epidural catheter tube is then passed in through the epidural needle. The needle itself is taken out and a small amount of local anaesthetic mixed with pain-killing drugs is injected down the catheter in liquid form.

It's very important to stay still throughout the procedure to ensure the needle is placed in the correct spot. This isn't easy to do, especially if your contractions are coming close together. But the anaesthetist will wait until the resting period between contractions to give the injection.

Sometimes it will take more than one attempt to complete the process because the spaces in between your back

Going all the way
It was long believed that an epidural should be allowed to wear off for the second stage of labour to avoid the need for forceps. However, research shows that this doesn't work – it just means the mother is in more pain than she needs to be. It's usually best to keep the epidural going (see References).

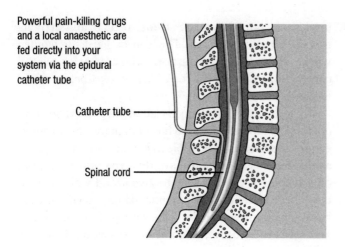

Powerful pain-killing drugs and a local anaesthetic are fed directly into your system via the epidural catheter tube

Catheter tube ———

Spinal cord ———

vertebrae are small and the anaesthetist has to be very sure that the needle has gone into exactly the right place.

An epidural's initial pain-relieving effects will wear off slightly and you will need topping up every couple of hours or so, which your midwife will be able to do. At many major centres they use a continuous infusion process. This is a low-level, steady stream of the drugs drip-fed into your system, which ensures that the effects don't wear off.

A few hospitals offer patient-controlled analgesia, whereby mothers in labour press a button to release more pain-killing drugs whenever they need to. Contrary to fears that people would overdose, in fact they tend to use far less if they can control it themselves.

How fast it works

A standard epidural takes about 20 minutes to set up and about another 10 to start working. However, because it can only be given by an anaesthetist, you may have to wait for anything from 10 minutes to a couple of hours if he or she is on call or shared with another hospital.

When you can, and can't, have it

This depends on how you are having your baby. If you are having your baby vaginally, you will usually need to wait

Failed attempt
If you are still feeling pain in a particular area half an hour after the epidural is put in, tell your midwife. The anaesthetist may need to be recalled and the epidural redone. This happens to as many as one in 30 women.

until your contractions are strong, regular and arriving every 5-10 minutes or so. This can be hard for women whose labour stops and starts, or who are having painful contractions on and off for a day or two before 'true' labour begins.

If you are having a planned Caesarean you can have an epidural as soon as you go to hospital. In the case of emergency Caesareans, it's possible to have an epidural as soon as the decision is made to have this type of delivery, but only if there is enough time to give it and wait for it to take effect. If there is any potential danger to you or your baby – perhaps your baby is becoming short of oxygen and needs to be delivered immediately – you might have a spinal instead or even a general anaesthetic, as these work straightaway.

Perhaps the most common reason for not being able to have an epidural is because an anaesthetist is not available. Smaller hospitals tend to share anaesthetists, and in larger hospitals it's possible that the anaesthetist is busy with another patient. Another reason is a shortage of midwives, as one needs to stay with you nearly all the time.

Women who are having their baby at home would not have the option of an epidural because the equipment needed is quite complicated and anaesthetists do not do home visits.

Home births

One in 50 British mothers has her baby at home. Pain-relief methods for home births include birthing pools, baths, warm showers, TENS, gas and air, massage, relaxation and visualisation, self-hypnosis, homeopathy, acupuncture, aromatherapy and reflexology.

From a medical point of view, epidurals are not given to women experiencing problems related to blood clotting and bleeding, such as placental abruption (when the placenta starts peeling away from the wall of the womb.) And if you're very near the second, or pushing, stage of labour, you may not be able to have an epidural because your doctor may feel that by the time an anaesthetist arrives and the epidural has been given, it will probably not have time to take effect before your baby is born.

Getting an epidural or spinal privately

Epidurals are available in 75% of UK hospitals with maternity units, but because there is no guarantee that you can definitely have one, some women prefer to pay for it privately.

However, to do so, you would almost certainly have to pay for medical care for the whole of your labour, not just for the services of an anaesthetist. A private pregnancy and childbirth care package costs anything from £3000-£8000 (sometimes more, depending on where you live and whether you need special care or additional tests). For this fee the same obstetrician will take care of you throughout your pregnancy, personally deliver your baby and do your postnatal check-up.

Private room charges are added on top, and they are about £500 or more per night. The latter can really add up, especially if this is your first baby and you want to stay in for several days. An NHS hospital will not usually let you stay for long since they now generally discharge women who have given birth within 24 hours if all's well. But most women need more recovery time than this. As recently as 1980, 10 days in an NHS hospital was standard.

It's important to realise, though, that while going private greatly *increases* your chances of having an epidural, it does not *guarantee* one because there may be good medical reasons why it would not be suitable or safe for you.

Epidurals and spinals – the pros

The following apply to all types of epidural and spinal pain-relieving techniques:

■ They are the strongest and most reliable methods of relieving labour pain. Women have been known to spend their labour on the phone, playing Scrabble, reading, watching TV or walking casually around the labour ward.

■ Because they reduce the physical stress of labour, they stop you becoming so tired.

■ Being in less pain will reduce your anxiety and help you become more relaxed, which in itself can help your labour go more smoothly and hurt less (see Breathing and relaxation, p122).

■ Some studies suggest that epidural-born babies arrive in better shape. This may be because the mother, being

What it costs
If you are having private medical care for your pregnancy and childbirth, you'll need to pay separately for a private anaesthetist to do your epidural. Expect to pay £400-£900.

more comfortable and in far less pain, produces fewer of the anxiety and stress hormones (adrenaline, noradrenaline and cortisol) that cross the placenta and affect her baby. It may also be because the blood pressure of mothers who have epidurals is not allowed to drop, so the supply of oxygen from their blood across the placenta to their baby is better and steadier.

'I'll never forget the relief I felt, and the look of relief on my partner's face, when the epidural kicked in'

- They are great for Caesareans. If you have your baby this way – unless it is a real emergency, which might necessitate a general anaesthetic – epidurals and spinals allow you to remain awake throughout and hold your baby straightaway.
- They are helpful if you need to have an assisted delivery with forceps or a ventouse. You won't feel any pain or discomfort when the instrument is inserted into your vagina and your baby is helped out.
- They are especially welcome if your labour is accelerated by drugs. The contractions drugs produce are very strong and arrive more frequently straightaway. Because you haven't experienced a gradual build-up to their intensity they can be more difficult to cope with.
- They are great for twins. If there is a delay between the deliveries (the second baby's delivery is often more complicated, too), an epidural helps prevent any deterioration in the condition of baby number two.

For epidurals alone – the pros:
- There is less chance of a splitting headache afterwards (these are more common with a spinal).
- Numbness comes on fairly slowly (within 15 minutes), so you have time to get used to the loss of sensation in your legs.

Epidurals and spinals – the cons
The following apply to all types of epidural and spinal pain-relieving techniques:
- There is no guarantee that you can have what you

want when the time comes, even if you made it plain that you would like an epidural or spinal well in advance.

■ About one in 20 women who have an epidural still experiences some pain.

■ You may experience uncontrollable shivering fits. Between one and two thirds of women experience these when they have an epidural (10-15% of women have them at some point during labour anyway, even without epidurals). However, these can often be treated very effectively.

■ They don't always work properly. It is quite a difficult procedure. The anaesthetist may at first put the needle in the wrong place and need to re-do it. Also, 'patchy' epidurals, which numb some areas but not others, or which are not initially effective, can happen to up to 13% of women. However, in large units with highly experienced anaesthetists, the figure is nearer 1%.

■ It's more likely to take longer to push your baby out. Epidurals inhibit your output of oxytocin, the hormone that makes your womb contract, which means your labour may slow down. To counteract this you may be given artificial oxytocin via a drip. And because you cannot feel your contractions, you cannot always co-ordinate your pushing effectively. It can help to watch the monitor or ask your midwife to rest her hand on your tummy and tell you when a contraction is peaking so you can time each push accordingly.

■ You are more likely have a forceps or ventouse delivery. If your labour slows down you may become too tired to push your baby out and so need an assisted delivery. Or if the pushing stage continues for too long, the constant powerful squeezing of the womb can cause your baby to become short of oxygen, and so it becomes a matter of urgency to get him out as soon as possible.

How long is too long to push? There is a fair bit of disagreement about this amongst the medical profession. But in practice it depends on how you are feeling and on your obstetrician's policy on the matter. Some doctors set the limit at an hour-and-a-half, while

Check ahead
Some maternity units do not have anaesthetists available 24 hours a day. If you are sure you want an epidural or spinal, phone your hospital a month or so ahead of your due date. The Anaesthetics Department can confirm whether or not they have 24-hour cover. If they don't, you may want to think about switching to a larger hospital.

others are willing to let a mother try for up to three hours if she is coping.

■ You may be more likely to need a Caesarean. A study of 896 women with 'uncomplicated pregnancies' at the UT Southwestern Medical Centre in Dallas (see References) found that on average the Caesarean rate among women who had epidurals tripled. However, it's also worth knowing that recent research in Sweden that looked at 85,691 epidural labours (see References), found that if women were given opioid (morphine-based) painkillers as well as an epidural, their chances of needing a Caesarean dropped sharply. If you'd like an epidural but are worried that it may lead to a Caesarean, ask your anaesthetist about the extra painkillers beforehand. Many are very approachable and they will probably know of the Swedish study.

■ You may suffer a splitting headache afterwards. This happens when fluid leaks out of a tiny tear in the dural membranes, which enclose the fluid circulating around the spinal cord, causing a slight drop in the pressure of the spinal fluid that bathes the spinal cord and brain. On average, fewer than 1% of women experience this.

■ The procedure is invasive, and some women just do not like the idea of a needle going deep into their spinal area, even though it only goes into a space between their vertebrae and does not touch the spinal cord.

■ They may make your baby jumpier and more fretful for a few days after birth, though this has not been proved conclusively.

■ With standard epidurals you have to stay in bed, either propped up on your side or in a reclining position. Having to stay like this for several hours can be extremely uncomfortable, and if you are semi-reclining you tend to slip downwards and need to have your position re-adjusted frequently to help avoid back pain and possible back problems after your baby's birth. This is not the best position to be in when you push your baby out either.

Headache after an epidural?

These are only supposed to last 24-48 hours, but if you're unlucky your headache can last up to a year or more. Do not suffer in silence, as these debilitating headaches do not go away on their own. Treatment is with a tiny blood patch that seals up the tear in the membranes that enclose the fluid around your spinal cord. This may need to be done more than once.

Epidurals and backache

Some research studies (see References) suggest that epidurals can virtually double your chances of suffering from backache after childbirth. The latest medical thinking is that post-epidural backaches are not so much caused by the needle nor the drugs it injects damaging the spinal area, but by the position the mother then spends the rest of her labour in. The fact that women who have a Caesarean with an epidural don't go on to experience more back problems than anyone else supports the theory that it's the labour position and not the needle itself that's to blame.

A professor of anaesthesia at St Thomas' Hospital, London, recalls how women who'd had an epidural would slip down the bed: 'We would give a woman her epidural, then I would come back a little later to see how she was getting on, to find out that, though she had initially been propped up well in bed, she had by now slipped downwards. This left a gap large enough to get my hand between her back and the angled back of the bed frame which was meant to be supporting it.'

Sitting for several hours in one position, with your back badly supported, puts great stress on back ligaments already softened by 40 weeks of pregnancy. As well as being miserably uncomfortable, this can increase the chances of damaging your back.

Prevention first, then cure

Research suggests that at least 50% of pregnant women experience some backache when they're pregnant. The worse it is, the more likely you are to have back problems after you've had your baby, too. Yet just a couple of visits to an osteopath or chiropractor in the last half of your pregnancy can help your back adjust to the growing demands of pregnancy and so avoid back pain. The practitioner can also help correct any new back trouble after your baby's birth.

Some osteopaths and chiropractors also have specialist training in paediatric and cranial techniques for newborn or very young babies, which can help ease many new baby problems, including colic and general fretfulness (see Resources for how to find a practitioner).

How to avoid back problems with an epidural

▪ Ask for a mobile epidural. You may not want to actually walk around that much – some women do, some don't – but you will be able to change positions easily. You will be able to lie down, squat, curl up on your side, kneel comfortably over a beanbag, or lean sideways on your partner's shoulder. Try sitting in a rocking chair, too (many maternity units now have them). Check with your maternity unit that it offers mobile epidurals, as most of the smaller units have only the standard variety.

If your hospital offers only standard epidurals:
▪ Ask for the foot of your bed to be tilted up a little to help stop you slipping down.
▪ Keep checking to see whether you have slipped – if you can place your hand in between your back and the bed, you have, so ask your midwife and/or partner to help you move up again.
▪ Ask your midwife to help you change positions every so often. Try sitting upright, with the soles of your feet together, lying on your side, or sitting propped up so you are semi-reclining, with a cushion or pillow supporting your knees.
▪ Use a beanbag for lower back support – it curves into you even better than a pillow, and it's bigger. Your labour ward may have one or you could bring in your own with you.
▪ If you are propped up, whether this is sideways or facing forward, check that the bend in your body is at hip level not waist level.
▪ If you don't mind being touched in labour, ask for your neck and shoulders to be massaged regularly as tension builds up here, leading to a bad headache and contributing to backache.

A spinal

A spinal is very similar to a standard epidural, except that the pain-killing drugs are injected directly into the bag of fluid surrounding your spine, rather than into the fat-filled space around it. This means that you feel the pain-relieving effect very quickly, usually within five minutes.

A spinal – the pros

- It is a very effective pain-reliever.
- It involves a simple, single-shot technique. After you've had a spinal, you may not feel another contraction for the whole of your labour.
- It is excellent for Caesarean deliveries, even some urgent ones, because it works so quickly. A spinal also leaves your mind clear and enables you to stay awake throughout the procedure, so you can hold your baby as soon as he is delivered.
- It uses a smaller amount of drugs than an epidural, and so less is transferred to your baby's system. A spinal baby may be less likely to be jittery in his first few days of life than an epidural baby.

A spinal – the cons

- It can be disconcerting to become this numb so fast.
- You are more likely to develop a severe headache than if you have a standard epidural.
- Your blood pressure may drop if a large amount of anaesthetic is used, which can make you feel sick, or actually vomit. However, this can be treated fast.

Mobile, or combined, epidural

Sometimes called a 'walking' epidural, this is a combination of a spinal and a standard epidural.

How fast it works

The spinal part provides pain relief within five minutes, and the epidural part provides ongoing pain relief without the total numbness a continuous spinal causes. Thus,

Freedom to move

If they are able to, women in labour change position an average of seven or eight times.

mobile epidurals enable you to retain enough sensation in your legs for you to change position freely and even walk around.

A mobile epidural is given in a similar way to a standard one, except that the anaesthetist uses two needles. One is placed in the fat-filled epidural space just outside the sac of fluid surrounding your spine; the other, longer one goes inside the first needle, through the epidural space, and slightly punctures the membrane (dura) that forms the sac of protective fluid around the spine.

If you have this form of pain relief you will need a midwife with you throughout your labour to monitor your blood pressure and pulse and your baby's heart rate.

Mobile epidural – the pros

- It is a very effective pain-reliever.
- You can move about, change position freely and even walk around.
- There is no need for a catheter in your bladder as you will be able to go to the toilet or use a bedpan.
- Very little of the anaesthetic drug is transferred to your baby, even in long labours of 16 hours or more.
- It can be given late in labour, when you are as much as 8-10cm dilated.

Mobile epidural – the cons

- It may cause itching. One study at Queen Charlotte's Hospital, London, found about 17% of women experienced this, but that it was seldom irritating enough to need treatment.
- You may have a severe headache afterwards, but this is less likely than if you have a spinal on its own.
- Because the spinal part of the procedure gives such quick pain relief, it can be harder for the anaesthetist to be sure that the epidural is in the right place.

The truth about paralysis

Some women feel instinctively wary about having an injection in their spine, and it doesn't help that the press fuels the fear with occasional stories about mothers being paralysed after they've had an epidural. But the chances of this happening are extremely remote – about one in a million.

What may occasionally happen is that a mother experiences minor nerve complications, such as pins and needles, or a small isolated numb patch, for anything from a few days to a few months after an epidural. This happens to about one in 10,000. More common is the possibility of having similar minor temporary neurological problems simply as a result of being pregnant and giving birth. These occur when the baby's head has been pressing particularly hard against a major nerve or nerves leading out of the pelvis, such as the femoral nerve, and it can take anything from a few weeks to a few months to repair.

Gas and air (Entonox)

Gas and air is a mixture of oxygen and nitrous oxide that you breathe in as you are having contractions. Sometimes referred to by its brand name, Entonox, it takes effect quickly, after just two or three breaths. It doesn't kill pain but rather dulls it by distancing you from it, making you feel light-headed and a bit drunk. Unlike other forms of pain relief, its effects wear off almost immediately when you stop breathing it in, and you can time its maximum effect to hit when a contraction peaks.

It works by depressing the action of the central nervous system, and by preventing the nerves in your spinal cord transmitting pain signals so well. For some women, breathing only 20% nitrous oxide can produce mild pain relief with slight sedation, but most women need higher concentrations. A mixture containing 50% is usually offered to women in labour.

Some people do not like its smell. Anaesthetists insist

'The Entonox experience is one of glorious indifference as inhibitions are unhinged. It is like the instantaneous effect of half a bottle of champagne with sobriety only four breaths away' the gas doesn't smell of anything, but many women describe it as sweetish and slightly sickly. Try having a breath or two of it when you look around the labour ward a couple of months before your baby is due. If you do notice its aroma, it will not come as a surprise to you when and if you have to use it. If you really dislike it, discuss other forms of pain relief with hospital staff.

Interestingly, many women who did not like the smell to begin with say that it didn't matter to them as their labour progressed and their contractions became stronger.

How you have it

The mixture of gases is either piped to an outlet on the wall above your bed, or provided in a wheeled cylinder that you can move around the room depending on what you are doing – lying on your bed, sitting in a chair, leaning over a beanbag or squatting on the floor. You take it in through a disposable plastic mouthpiece (a new one is used for every mother) that you hold to your mouth or clench between your teeth. A 'demand' valve on the cylinder ensures the gas only starts flowing when you breathe in. You breathe out through the mouthpiece, too.

'It really gave me something positive and helpful to do during the contractions instead of just waiting until they had gone away. This helped stop me tensing up each time one came'

It's a good idea to take only four or five deep breaths of the gas per contraction. If you take in too much the effect will carry on after the contraction is over, which may make you miss the beginning of the next one. When you are inhaling the gas you must not walk or stand because it can make you feel dizzy. But because the effects of the gas wear off so fast, you can move around freely again once you've stopped inhaling.

Because gas and air can make you feel light-headed, you may find it difficult to use it properly or work out what your midwife is saying. As one female anaesthetist who has had three babies put it: 'Did she say breathe into your mask, push into your bottom, or do you care anyway?'

When you can, and can't, have it

You can use gas and air at almost any time during labour, but it is generally used towards the end of the first stage, when contractions are regular and strong, rather than earlier on, when many women like to move around. And if you start using the gas early on, and continue to use it for a long time, it may make you feel sick and dizzy.

Gas and air can also be used in the second stage of labour, when you deliver your baby. However, some obstetricians feel it distracts women from pushing their baby out as efficiently as they would do if they had no pain relief. Talk about this with your obstetrician and midwife beforehand. If they advise against it but you find when the time comes that you cannot manage without it, and provided there is no medical reason why you should not have it, keep using the gas and air – you are the one having the baby and the pain, not them.

You may also find it useful when your midwife or obstetrician carries out vaginal examinations. These are done to see how far your cervix has dilated so staff can tell how close you are to delivering your baby. These examinations are done regularly throughout your labour and, because you will be very sensitive in that area during childbirth, they can be quite uncomfortable, though not as a rule painful as long as you relax and the person examining you is gentle and skilled. The examinations may be less uncomfortable if your midwife carries them out while you are lying on your left side, rather than flat on your back. This is also better for your baby as it helps maintain a good blood supply to the placenta.

Gas and air can also be used to supplement an epidural that is wearing off, or if you need to have stitches to repair a tear or episiotomy after your baby is born. And it's a handy form of pain relief if you are having a rapid delivery since there's not often enough time to use any other method.

You will not be able to use gas and air if you are very drowsy or not fully conscious.

Using gas and air
To get the maximum effect from gas and air, start to breathe it in just as the pain of your contraction is beginning, then stop at the pain's peak.

How effective it is

About 75% of women in labour use gas and air at some point. But while it works well for some, it doesn't for others. The National Birthday Trust survey in 1990, which looked at the effectiveness and popularity of all available methods of pain relief in labour, found that eight out of 10 women thought gas and air was either 'good' or 'very good'. However, other research suggests it is of no more use than a placebo (dummy) treatment.

> 'I think gas and air should be tried before things get out of hand so you know how to use it and how it makes you feel'

Gas and air – the pros

- It works almost immediately.
- It is under your own control, so whenever you feel you need more you just breathe it in. Because you are in charge of the mouthpiece yourself, you are unlikely to overdose.
- It is widely available – even ambulances have it. And it can also be used if you are having your baby at home.
- It can be helpful. Although it does not provide complete pain relief, it will at least take the edge off.
- It can be used when there is no time for any other form of pain relief to work.
- Between breaths of gas and air you can move about a certain amount (just around your room or cubicle rather than up and down the hospital corridors). But you must sit down well-supported while inhaling it. It also allows you to get into different positions that will help your labour (leaning over a beanbag or the back of chair, or squatting while being supported).
- You can use other forms of pain relief with it. These include all self-help and natural methods, such as yoga, self-hypnosis, breathing and relaxation, autogenic training, massage and visualisation. Your midwife may let you use it in a birthing pool or bath as long as you have someone with you in case you start to feel groggy and slip under the water (some water birth purists say

that the water itself should be enough – and for many women, it is). TENS, too, can be used with gas and air as they don't interfere with each other.

■ It can be used while waiting for an epidural, which is worth knowing as the delay between requesting an epidural and feeling its effects can be at least 30

'It went well with the breathing methods of relaxation I had been taught in my antenatal classes – it gave them extra power'

minutes, usually more. You can also use gas and air at the same time as an epidural, if the latter has missed an area and you are still in some pain, or has been allowed to wear off a bit in the second stage so that you can push better.

Gas and air – the cons

■ You might not like the smell/taste of the gas, especially if you are feeling sick, which is quite common for at least part of labour.

■ Your baby may be slightly affected if you inhale the gas for several hours on end and start over-breathing (breathing rapidly and shallowly), as this can reduce your, and therefore your baby's, oxygen supply.

■ The nitrous oxide in the gas can cause changes to a particular enzyme, which in theory could affect your baby's metabolism, but this has never been found to happen to a great enough extent to make any difference.

■ You may feel dizzy and disorientated, especially if you are inhaling too much. If this happens, stop for a while, until the feeling passes.

■ It can give you mild amnesia afterwards.

■ It's not a very strong pain-reliever.

General anaesthetic

A general anaesthetic (GA) produces rapid and total unconsciousness. When used in labour it is not a method of pain relief in the usual sense, yet because it causes rapid loss of consciousness it can stop you feeling any pain at all. GAs are generally used in labour for emergency Caesareans only, when there is not enough time to set up an epidural or even a fast-acting spinal (p63). And if the placenta is not delivered in the normal way during the third stage of labour, and is still inside the womb, a GA is necessary to surgically remove it.

A GA will last for as long as the Caesarean operation lasts, usually about 45 minutes. Depending on how much anaesthetic is used, you could be awake very soon after the operation is over. It will then take 24-48 hours to recover from most of its aftereffects.

How you have it

A GA is given as a combination of a drug that is injected into a vein in the back of your hand to send you to sleep, then a gas that you breathe in to keep you sedated. After you've fallen asleep the anaesthetist's assistant will press their fingers just below your larynx, or Adam's apple. This is to make sure that, as your muscles relax, the contents of your stomach don't rise up into your mouth, where they will be in danger of entering your lungs as the anaesthetist puts a breathing tube down your airway. This tube will remain in place for the rest of the operation. It is linked to a ventilator that 'breathes' for you throughout, making sure you receive the right amount of oxygen for yourself and your baby, and the right amount of anaesthetic gas to keep you asleep.

Throughout the operation the anaesthetist will continually monitor your blood pressure, heart rate and levels of oxygen and carbon dioxide. When the surgery is finished the flow of anaesthetic will be turned off and you will be gently brought back to consciousness.

When you can, and can't, have it

There are very few times when you cannot have a GA if one is needed. You won't be able to have one if you've recently had a large meal because of the risk of vomiting or inhaling the contents of your stomach into your lungs. But it's unlikely that a woman in labour would have had that much to eat anyway. It may also not be suitable for some women who have severe heart or breathing problems.

General anaesthetic – the pros
■ It can enable invasive but life-saving procedures for a mother, her baby, or both to be carried out almost immediately when necessary.
■ It gives total pain relief.
■ It works very fast.

General anaesthetic – the cons
For you:
■ Women who have had a Caesarean under GA may feel disappointed and distressed afterwards. Some report feeling that they were not there at all, that they have no real way of being sure the baby is theirs, and that they have missed something very important and precious – awareness of their baby's birth. Others say they felt very disappointed they were unable to give birth to their child naturally. (If you would like someone to talk to about this, or any other aspect of Caesarean birth, such as how to be up and about as quickly as possible afterwards, or the easiest ways to breastfeed, contact the Caesarean Support Network – see Resources.)
■ You and your baby may be sleepy and feel sick or groggy for many hours afterwards, which can make it more difficult to bond and establish breastfeeding.
■ It can take weeks to recover totally, and some women report feeling more tired and lethargic than usual, with less mental sharpness, for several weeks. This is not just the effect of the operation itself, as people who have had minimally invasive surgery, such as a laparoscopy (a look inside the pelvis or abdomen through a keyhole-size incision that only requires a single repair stitch but is done under GA), say the same.
■ If the procedure is carried out as an emergency, it can be very alarming for the mother and her partner.
■ There is a risk of infection and thrombosis.

For your baby:

▪ It can affect your baby, but by how much remains a subject of debate. You'll probably be told that your baby will not show any ill effects after 24-48 hours. However, some mothers have said their babies were more irritable, less responsive than expected, and only wanted to suckle for short periods until they were several weeks old. This meant they were more difficult to care for, and that it was harder to get them feeding well and happily, especially if they were being breastfed.

▪ The GA may affect your baby's ability to breathe unaided, which means he may need additional help. This may also have something to do with your baby not having gone through ordinary labour. Specialists in fetal (unborn baby) medicine suggest that the way your contractions squeeze your baby helps stimulate him to breathe, and if he does not have that stimulus he may find breathing alone more difficult at first.

Waking up during a Caesarean section under GA

You may have heard stories about people waking up while on the operating table, unable to let medical staff know they are conscious, and suffering pain and distress both during and after their Caesarean. Although women may 'surface' very occasionally, the awareness experienced is usually fleeting, and almost never takes the form of pain.

About 200 of the 40,000 (1 in 200) mothers who have the operation under GA each year in the UK experience a very slight degree of consciousness at some point during the procedure (see References). However, all they are likely to be aware is being physically manipulated or hearing noises like their baby crying, the ticking of anaesthetic machinery, or snatches of the medical staff's conversations.

Becoming wakeful while under GA is more likely to happen during a Caesarean than during any other sort of operation because the initial amount of anaesthetic used is lower than normal so as not to affect the baby. But once the baby has been lifted out of his mother's womb, the dosage is then increased and the chance of waking drops.

A study carried out by St James' Hospital, Leeds, in 1991 shows that waking under GA happens less often than it used to because anaesthetists are increasingly customising doses of anaesthetic drugs rather than sticking to rigid guidelines.

Having your baby by Caesarean

A Caesarean section is a safe, common operation, and one in five babies in Britain is now born this way. Yet because it is carried out so often, it's easy to lose sight of the fact that it is also major abdominal surgery, which will take about three months to recover from sufficiently to be able to get on with your daily life, and up to a year or more to get over completely.

To perform a Caesarean your obstetrician makes an incision through your abdominal wall, then your womb, and lifts your baby out. This may be done under heavy local anaesthetic (an epidural or a spinal) or under light general anaesthetic, planned well in advance for a particular day or carried out as an emergency procedure.

Caesareans have their own section in this book, as they do need specific types of pain relief.

Elective (planned) Caesareans

If you are having a baby by elective (planned) Caesarean section, you do not need to wait for labour to begin. In fact, you will not go into labour at all and so will not have any labour pains. Instead, you will be booked in to hospital to have the operation done on a specific day. Reasons for an elective Caesarean include:

■ Your previous baby or babies were born this way. If you want to have your next baby vaginally, discuss it with your obstetrician beforehand. About one third of expectant mothers who have previously had a Caesarean go on to give birth in the usual way, so if there is no medical reason to prevent it, you could go into labour as normal and see how things progress.

Sign of the times
One in five babies in Britain is now born by Caesarean section. Yet as recently as 1989 it was only one in 20.

However, if problems do develop, the staff will intervene and you will need another Caesarean. The Caesarean Support Network gives information and encouragement to women who have had one or more babies this way and wish to avoid another Caesarean (see Resources).

■ Placenta praevia. This means that your placenta is lying low down in your womb, perhaps blocking the opening where your baby should come out.

■ If your baby is lying in an unusual way. If some part of your baby other than the top of his head – perhaps his bottom or feet – is against your cervix, it may be difficult for him to leave your womb. When a baby is lying with his back across the exit from the womb – a 'transverse lie' – he cannot be born vaginally.

■ When your baby's head is too large to pass through your pelvis easily. Obstetricians and midwives call this cephalo-pelvic disproportion. Sometimes it is obvious that this is going to be a problem, but at other times the medical staff are not quite sure, and will suggest you have a trial labour, where you try to give birth yourself for a while. If your labour does not progress well and your baby's head is clearly not coming down into the birth canal, you would have a Caesarean.

■ Your labour isn't progressing. Experienced staff should be able to tell the difference between a labour that is naturally slow but progressing at its own pace, and one that is hardly moving along at all and needs major help. Unless your baby is showing signs of distress, or you are becoming exhausted, they will probably try hastening your labour gently at first, perhaps with prostaglandin pessaries. If that doesn't work, they may try an artificial oxytocin drip, which can produce sharper and more effective contractions. If that doesn't work well either, they will give you a Caesarean.

■ Certain health problems that you may have. These include:

　■ Active genital herpes (when the herpes sores are actually visible, not when they have disappeared). If your baby is born vaginally when you have an active herpes sore, you can pass the infection on to him.

- Diabetes, as this can mean that your baby will be larger than usual. The average weight of a full-term baby is about 7lbs, but if you are diabetic there will be extra sugar in your bloodstream, and this will have passed to your baby throughout your pregnancy, making him larger than usual – more than 10lbs is not unusual. One in 50 women develops diabetes just during pregnancy – in Asian women it's nearer one in 10. This is called gestational diabetes and it subsides after childbirth.
- Very high blood pressure.
- Full-blown eclampsia, which may result in you having convulsions and your baby being born prematurely.
- If you are HIV positive. There is less chance of passing on the infection to your baby during the birth if he is delivered by Caesarean. According to the UK Public Health Laboratory Service, there are several things that you and your obstetrician can do to 'almost eliminate' the risk of your baby being infected, too. The main ones are taking antiviral drugs in the last three months of your pregnancy, having your Caesarean using laser surgery for what is known as a bloodless Caesarean, and bottle-feeding rather than breastfeeding.
- Not wanting an epidural or spinal. Most Caesareans are done using one or the other, but some mothers are not happy about the thought of being awake throughout the operation, or of having an injection in their spine. It is really important that you are happy with how you choose to have your Caesarean, both as it is being done and afterwards, so if a planned one is on the cards, now is the time to talk to your obstetrician about any concerns. Tell him or her how you feel, and ask about the option of a general anaesthetic instead. Modern general anaesthetics do have fewer side effects on both mother and baby than in the past but, if possible, it is better to avoid a GA.

How an elective Caesarean is done

First, the staff might clip your pubic hair. Then you might be given a suppository to empty your bladder and bowel, because once the epidural is working you will no longer have control over either. You will also have a catheter put into your bladder to drain it, and a drip in your arm to help prevent falls in blood pressure.

If time allows, talk to your obstetrician about where you would prefer the scar to be. The incision is usually made horizontally just below the bikini line, but there may be medical reasons why it's necessary to do a vertical one from your pubic area to your belly button.

If you are having an epidural or spinal, the staff will set up the equipment. If not, you will be given a general anaesthetic (p79). Where an epidural or spinal is used, a screen will be placed across your waist so you cannot easily see the operation. However, if you would like to watch, the staff can hold up a mirror for you. Your obstetrician will probably give an encouraging running commentary for you anyway, explaining what is being done and how it is all going.

After the incision is made the amniotic fluid will be sucked out (you will hear this as a gurgling or sucking sound) and your obstetrician will lift your baby out, pressing down on your abdomen as he does so. Many women say they experienced a rummaging feeling, 'as if someone was doing their washing in my stomach', while others report sensations of pulling and stretching. If you have had an epidural or spinal, you will be able to see your baby being lifted out, hear his first cry and hold him straightaway.

You will then be given an injection to speed up the expulsion of your placenta, after which the incision will be stitched. The birth itself takes less than 10 minutes, but the careful sewing-up afterwards may take 40. You do not need any additional pain relief for this because your epidural will still be working.

If your Caesarean is done under GA you won't remember anything when you wake up. Some women feel uncomfortable about coming round from the anaesthetic and then being handed a baby and told it is theirs. If you feel this might worry you, it may help if your partner (if allowed to be present) or one of the staff takes a Polaroid photo of the baby being lifted from your womb.

Emergency (unplanned) Caesareans

An emergency Caesarean section is one that, instead of being planned and discussed well in advance, becomes necessary at what may be very short notice, when you are already in labour. It may be needed for any of the reasons mentioned on p83-85 or because your placenta is peeling away from the womb wall, preventing it from keeping your baby supplied with all the oxygen-rich blood he needs. However, one of the most common additional reasons is that your baby is in distress, usually because he is not getting enough oxygen. This can happen as a result of:
■ The physical stress that labour places on your baby, as well as on you yourself.
■ You baby's umbilical cord, which should carry his supply of oxygen, becoming partly or totally squashed so little or no oxygenated blood can get through to him.

Medical staff can tell if your baby might be in distress if his heartbeat becomes rapid (this is detected through a monitoring device placed on your stomach), or if there is meconium (the baby's first bowel movement) in the amniotic fluid. Meconium can be seen quite clearly if your waters have broken because it is greenish so it shows up well. If an unborn baby becomes short of oxygen in the womb, he gets frightened, and the fear makes him empty his bowels into the amniotic fluid (your waters) surrounding him.

Setting up an epidural can take some time, so if your baby needs to be born straightaway to avoid possible harm, you will be given a spinal or a general anaesthetic. This means the operation can begin within just a few minutes, as opposed to the 30 minutes or more you would have to wait for an epidural. The exception is if you have already been given an epidural for pain relief during your

Mirror image
If you don't want to see anything at all of your Caesarean, avoid catching the reflection in the mirrored lights above the operating table. Concentrate on your partner, if he is with you, or on talking to one of the staff instead.

Be safe
If you are allergic to a particular type of local anaesthetic, tell your obstetrician or midwife so it won't be given to you.

labour, and the necessary tube is already set up. If this is the case, the anaesthetist can use the tube to give you a much heavier dose of local anaesthetic, one that will numb you totally from the waist down so you won't feel a thing.

There is a small possibility that an epidural may not work fully, but in almost all cases this becomes obvious before the operation begins, in which case the staff will use an extra method of pain relief as well.

Paracervical block

This is a local anaesthetic injection given on either side of your cervix, and it provides good pain relief in just a few minutes. It is usually used at the end of the first stage of labour, when the dilation of your cervix can be particularly uncomfortable. In fact, you can only have it once your cervix is 6cm dilated, so it is not an option for early labour.

Its effects usually last for 30-60 minutes and if the injections are timed right they will provide you with pain relief into the second stage of labour, when you are pushing your baby out. It can also be used if you need an assisted delivery using forceps. However, it is rarely used in the UK these days – it's more common in the USA.

Paracervical block – the pros
- It can be effective.
- It works fast.

Paracervical block – the cons
- It's not effective, or even available, for all stages of labour.
- The pain relief it provides does not last very long.
- It can affect your baby's heart rate, causing it to slow. This may be either because of the direct effect of the anaesthetic on the blood vessels supplying your womb, or because of the delayed effect on those same blood vessels, which go into spasm later on when the anaesthetic has been absorbed into your bloodstream.

Pethidine

Pethidine is a synthetic, narcotic drug similar to morphine. It is also commonly known as meperidine, and by the brand names Dolantin, Dolosal and Demerol. A strong painkiller, it works within about 15 minutes, usually hitting its peak within half an hour, but it also makes you feel drowsy and distant.

In the National Birthday Trust's survey in 1990 only about one quarter of the women who used pethidine thought it was 'very good'. It used to be very popular but is used less these days because many maternity units now feel it isn't that helpful after all, that it can make women feel disorientated and out of control of their labours, and that it can also affect the baby. Some hospitals have even stopped using it. Despite this, at least one third of British women in labour still have it.

Interestingly, some midwives seem to feel pethidine is more helpful than the women who actually use it do. This may be because it makes 80% of women who use it sleepy. If a woman in labour is making little fuss because she is drowsy (even though she may still be in considerable discomfort) an observer might well think that she is in less pain than before she was given the pethidine.

How you have it

Your midwife or obstetrician can prescribe pethidine for you. It will usually be injected into the muscle of your thigh or buttock. It may also be given intravenously (injected straight into a vein), but this would only be done if you needed an emergency procedure that required immediate strong pain relief but did not merit a general anaesthetic, such as an emergency forceps delivery.

In larger hospitals it's sometimes possible to have pethidine via patient-controlled analgesia, where you give yourself a small dose whenever you need it using a computer-controlled syringe pump.

How fast it works

A standard injection takes effect within 15 minutes and

provides pain relief for about two or three hours before wearing off. If it is given intravenously it will work straightaway for about half an hour then wear off. However, your baby may feel the effects of pethidine for several days. It used to be the case that one or two standard doses were given to women having a normal labour, but midwives now often customise doses for individual women. If you have a smaller dose, the effect will be gentler and not last as long.

When you can, and can't, have it

In the past midwives felt that pethidine should be given in early labour so that it had the least effect on the baby. However, the most recent thinking is quite the opposite. It's now thought that an early dose would give the drug more time to cross the placenta and build up in the baby's own tissues.

He would then have to eliminate it from his body himself in the first few days following his birth, and until he did, the drug could make him sleepy and irritable and affect his ability to breastfeed and breathe unaided.

Obstetricians now usually suggest giving the drug very late on in labour, not too long before the actual birth. However, because it is difficult to judge exactly how far away from delivery a mother is (plus the fact that maternity staff now feel pethidine is not that helpful to women in labour after all), an increasing number of maternity units seldom use it.

'I think pethidine helped me to relax. It did not relieve the pain though. What it did do was make me mentally dopey and out of control and less concerned about it'

You won't be able to have pethidine if your baby is premature because it can affect a baby's breathing, and premature babies tend to have more trouble breathing unaided at first anyway. Nor will you be able to have it if you have breathing-related problems such as acute asthma, chronic bronchitis and emphysema, or severe liver disease, as your body won't be able to break down the drug easily, or if you are taking monoamine oxidase inhibitors (MAOI) for depression.

Pethidine – the pros

■ It can be a mood enhancer. Some women feel euphoric and high, distanced from the pain, as if they are floating above it.

■ It is useful if your contractions are painful but they are not having much effect and your cervix is dilating extremely slowly. Because pethidine makes you sleepy, some women are able to doze for as long as four hours, then wake up to find they are in good established labour at last and are able to manage the rest of their labour with renewed energy.

Pethidine – the cons

For you:

■ It makes about one in three women feel sick, and a few actually vomit. Some women feel nauseous during their transition phase and are sick anyway, so any sickness caused by pethidine would be in addition to this. Therefore, the drug is usually given with anti-sickness medication. To be on the safe side, check with your midwife that she is definitely going to give you anti-nausea medication, too.

■ Some women are simply knocked sideways by it.

■ The sleepiness can have a down side, because waking up to find you are in full-throttle labour can be a shock.

■ The sedative effect can slow down labour. As one partner put it: 'Pethidine gave her pain relief but it brought labour to a standstill.'

■ Some women (about 5%) may experience a drop in blood pressure. It is important to tell your midwife or obstetrician immediately if you feel any dizziness or tingling in your fingers and toes. Temporary drops in blood pressure can be countered easily if you have a drip for a while.

■ It can cause amnesia. If the drug is given towards the end of labour you may have no memory of your baby's birth. This is not usual, but when it happens it can be very upsetting.

■ You may feel disorientated. Rather than being agreeably

Minimising the risk
If pethidine is given just before you give birth – within half an hour or so of delivery – it may not go across the placenta and affect your baby at all.

high you could feel as though you are unpleasantly drunk and that your labour is out of control.

■ A small number of women (less than 1%) may suffer severe disorientation and hallucinations. These may be pleasant but they can also be alarming. One woman we interviewed thought she was in a prison hospital and that the obstetricians were going to take her baby away as soon as he had been born.

'I was very disappointed with pethidine as I could not think straight and could not do as I was told'

■ You may not be allowed to eat anything to keep your energy levels up.

For your baby:

■ It may temporarily affect your baby's ability to breathe well. This is barely noticeable to the naked eye, but it can certainly make a difference to the child himself from the moment he is born.

■ He may be rather sleepy and unresponsive for a few days after his birth, until the pethidine is out of his system. This may sound as if it's no bad thing – many mothers wouldn't mind a peaceful baby who sleeps a good deal. But this sleepiness can also affect your baby's ability to feed and suckle and this can cause problems for mothers who are trying to breastfeed, especially if they are first-time mothers. A baby who is sleepy and less alert at first may also be a little more difficult to bond with than a more responsive baby.

■ He may be more fretful and more easily startled than he would otherwise be. And an irritable, jumpy baby who cries a lot and is not easily comforted can make the first few days after childbirth really difficult for a new mother, and she may start losing confidence in herself.

Pudendal block

This is a local anaesthetic injection given just below your pelvis. Used in the second stage of labour, it deadens the feeling around the perineum when the baby is being delivered. It is more likely to be used when a baby is arriving bottom-first, or if forceps or a ventouse is needed to help him out.

Nerve blocks are used in about 10-20% of all births but their use is decreasing steadily, and many trainee obstetricians are no longer even being taught how to do them.

Pudendal block – the pros
- It acts quickly, within just a few minutes.
- It can be very effective.

Pudendal block – the cons
- It does not always help because the injection does not block all the major nerves going to the perineum.
- Your pudendal nerve is close to the blood vessels that supply your baby in the womb and if large amounts of anaesthetic are used your baby's heart rate could be affected. This, however, is not likely to happen as the person giving the injection will limit the amounts of drug he or she uses.

Natural Methods

Western society is now using more natural medicines and therapies than ever before to help cure its ills and stay healthy. Many of these are 'complementary medicines', which means they can be successfully used alongside conventional medicine. Therapies that are used instead of conventional medicine are now known as 'alternative'.

Natural therapies seem to be especially helpful for conditions that can be partially stress-related, such as heart disease, asthma, eczema, premenstrual syndrome and stomach-related problems such as ulcers and irritable bowel syndrome, and for back problems and other musculo skeletal conditions. Chiropractors and osteopaths, who are the most popular complementary practitioners in the UK, often treat the latter. These therapies are also helpful in dealing with many types of pain, from the nagging low level sort (caused, for example, by very mild arthritis) to severe and acute distress.

In Europe studies suggest that between one third and one half of us have used some form of complementary

Getting the thumbs up

It's not just the consumers who use complementary medicine who rate it. One third of British midwives now use it in their practices (see References), and a recent study by the Royal College of GPs found that six out of 10 trainee family doctors want to train in a form of complementary medicine alongside their ordinary medical studies.

medicine, although different therapies may top the list in different countries. A Consumers' Association survey found that three out of the top five most popular therapies in the UK are homeopathy, aromatherapy and acupuncture, all of which can be useful in dealing with pain relief in labour. About 80% of Britons have used complementary medicine.

In the USA a 1993 survey found that one in three people had used complementary medicine, and predicted this would rise to one in two by 2000. Tellingly, even several hard-bitten medical insurance companies in the USA are now covering certain complementary medicines if the treatment is recommended by a doctor. In Australia nearly half the population is said to use, or have used, at least one natural remedy.

Integrated Medicine – a step forward

During the past few years progressive doctors in the orthodox medical establishment have begun to encourage the fusion of natural therapies and conventional modern medicine – two very different sorts of healing – calling it Integrated Medicine (IM).

IM is increasingly being seen as the way forward because it takes the best from both sides and offers patients a carefully integrated new form of healthcare. It is being taken so seriously in some quarters that in 2001 the influential Royal College of Physicians, a traditional British medical organisation not known for its radicalism, hosted a major international conference in London alongside the USA's powerful Institute of Health. The subject was how the IM approach is already being applied in research and patient care on both sides of the Atlantic, and how to develop it further.

But if natural therapies are so popular, how come they aren't used more often in childbirth? Well, perhaps they are. Accurate information about how much complementary medicine is used in labour isn't available because hospitals often don't record its use. They only have to record the use of drug-based pain relief, since they are officially accountable for what gets used from their drug cabinets. They do not have to record what women bring onto the ward themselves, whether that might be a reflexologist or some homeopathic remedies.

Drug-based pain relief versus natural

According to official figures, about 20% of women in labour have an epidural, about 75% use gas and air, and about 33% use pethidine. A small percentage uses natural methods, such as birthing pools and TENS, and complementary therapies, such as reflexology, aromatherapy and acupuncture.

Although these figures partly take into account the fact that women often use more than one form of pain relief during labour (gas and air, for instance, is used before or alongside many other forms), they don't take into account the full extent to which complementary therapies and natural methods are used alongside conventional forms of pain relief.

Natural methods on offer at hospitals

There are several possible reasons why drug-based methods of pain relief are used more often than natural methods. For a start, drug-based methods are far more widely available in hospitals. Nearly all hospitals offer epidurals and pethidine, but while many have a birthing pool, a smaller proportion has TENS. Acupuncture and aromatherapy are only offered in a few areas of the country, in specific progressive hospitals. And even though there are five totally homeopathic hospitals in the NHS system dealing with general medicine, homeopathy isn't offered on state-funded labour wards at all.

If you ask about the methods of pain relief available at your hospital, you will probably be given printed information on the various drugs on offer and perhaps a bit about relaxation and TENS. But it is a rare unit that will tell you about any natural methods, too, because, with a few notable exceptions, they don't know much about the subject.

Information is power
Not everyone knows that complementary therapies can be strong enough to help with something as powerful as labour pain. And even if they are aware of the benefits, they may not know where to get more information.

The onus is on you

Drug-based (pharmacological) methods of pain relief are provided free in the NHS. Whereas, apart from water, relaxation and possibly TENS, you will probably need to arrange any drug-free methods yourself and pay for them privately. With some of them, such as self-hypnosis, relaxation, visualisation and autogenic training, you also need to practise them for a while before you need them in labour.

The cost can be off-putting – having a complementary practitioner, such as a homeopath, with you in labour can cost a couple of hundred pounds. However, it's possible to cut costs considerably by learning techniques from books, workshops and special courses that may be run by midwives and complementary practitioners, and by getting one-to-one advice from a professional therapist.

Natural does not mean weaker

Drugs are seen as a strong and effective way of killing labour pain. Natural therapies are seen as gentler, with fewer or no side effects. But because they work more subtly, many people feel they cannot possibly be powerful enough.

Yet the available figures for several complementary methods tell a different story. For instance, research on acupuncture for childbirth (p102) suggests that the pain relief it provides is 'good' or 'very good' for about 60% of the mothers who use it. The studies indicate it can reduce the pain by one to two thirds, and that it also has the added bonus of making labours about one third shorter. Studies on aromatherapy (p108), autogenic training (p117) and self-hypnosis (see hypnotherapy, p143) suggest these methods have similar effects.

If these figures are to be believed, they imply that these complementary therapies are actually more effective at relieving labour pain than the most popular drugs hospital maternity units use. For example, only about 25% of mothers who use pethidine (offered by almost every hospital) consider it 'good' or 'very good'. And as for gas and air, though some research says that 80% of the women

Knowing what will work
While it is difficult to say in advance how much any form of pain relief (drug or natural) is going to help you, natural methods may be generally less predictable than drugs. Statistical records for drugs mean that their success or failure rate is easier to put a figure on – though there is no guarantee that they will suit you or work for you.

who use it find it 'good' or 'very good', other studies show that it is of no more use than a placebo treatment. And neither method will make your labour any quicker.

Side effects

Of the most commonly used pain-relieving drugs in labour, it is now widely accepted that pethidine can have several negative side effects for both mother and baby. Gas and air has a few, but they are pretty minor (dizziness, disorientation and confusion) and tend to wear off quickly. Epidurals and spinals, the most effective forms of pain relief, have several potential side effects, some of them quite severe, such as long-term splitting headaches (p70).

Yet the research that exists for natural therapies suggests that there are virtually no side effects when they are used to relieve pain in childbirth. And when there are any, they are uncommon and tend be minor, such as a temporary skin rash if one of the aromatherapy oils disagrees with you.

It is likely that if more information were available on how complementary therapies help in labour, more mothers would use them.

Using complementary therapies in hospital

If you are having your baby in hospital and would like to have a professional complementary therapist (say, an acupuncturist or homeopath) with you during your labour, check with the Head of Midwifery Services several months before your due date that the hospital is happy for you to do this.

Some hospitals will be fine about it, some won't. It depends on the policy of the midwifery unit and on your consultant, who will still be legally responsible for the welfare of you and your baby should anything go wrong.

If the hospital is reluctant, argue your case. Ask them, tactfully, if they have come across any clinical research that backs up the therapy's use in childbirth (see References for some useful ones as a start). Offer to show them what you have found if they are interested. Check that your therapist has comprehensive professional insurance and

It's not a class thing
It is often suggested that it is mostly middle-class women who are interested in natural methods of pain relief. However, a study of 700 women in six maternity units in Southeast England in 1993 showed that social class and occupation make no difference. Most mothers from all classes wanted to avoid having to use pain-killing drugs.

registration, and tell the hospital about this. Mention other hospitals that allow complementary therapy on the labour wards or in other departments (quite often the oncology unit and cardiac and pain clinics).

If your hospital still says no, try to find a more open-minded one. Community midwives can be a good source of information for this, as they should know the attitude local hospitals and their consultants take towards complementary medicine. It's worth knowing, too, that different obstetricians in the same hospital will have different policies, and some may be more sympathetic to this type of pain relief than others.

Anaesthetists (doctors with highly specialised training in pain relief and anaesthesia) are often very approachable and happy to answer questions from pregnant women about all aspects of pain relief. If you would like to talk to one about complementary therapies, or any other aspect of pain relief for childbirth, ask at one of your antenatal appointments. They may also know of one of their colleagues in a nearby hospital who has an interest in complementary medicine, or they may be sympathetic to it themselves and prepared to have a word with any sceptical consultant obstetricians on your behalf.

Contact help groups and information organisations. The Independent Midwives Association (IMA), whose members are NHS-trained midwives who work privately, your local National Childbirth Trust and local Active Birth class tutors may be able to tell you which hospitals welcome complementary therapists.

And ask the therapists themselves. If they have an interest in taking care of pregnant women, they might well know which maternity units are worth approaching. Some of the more liberal-minded hospitals may well be private, though, and a privately managed pregnancy and birth can cost £3000-£8000 or more.

The danger of not having permission

Do not simply arrive at the hospital in labour with your complementary therapist unless you've cleared it with the

Bonding issue

Women in labour in Japan today are unlikely to be offered much in the way of pain relief because the Japanese still believe that the pain of childbirth helps mothers bond more powerfully with their newborns.

hospital and got their agreement in writing. Bring that agreement with you to show the labour ward staff, as this may be the first they've heard of it. Otherwise, it's possible that your therapist will not be allowed onto the labour ward at all unless it's just as a friend or birth companion. There have even been cases of women being told to choose between the therapist and their partner.

If your therapist is refused admission, you will still have to pay her bill, or at the very least a cancellation fee. But, worst of all, you will be without the type of pain relief you want and have taken such trouble to arrange.

Why hospitals say 'No' to therapists

There are several reasons why hospitals might have a problem with a complementary therapist coming into the maternity unit with you:

■ Some are concerned about the therapist's insurance status in case of medical complications. Check that your therapist has the necessary professional insurance to cover her to give pain relief to women in labour. Let the hospital know that he or she has it.

■ The maternity staff may not know much about complementary medicine, or may not be keen on it in principle.

■ They may understandably want to see evidence of the therapy's safety and effectiveness in the sort of standard, extensive clinical trials that they're used to seeing for drug treatments. However, there are not many of these supporting the use of complementary therapies in childbirth, compared with the hundreds of trials that have been done on drug-based methods of pain relief. And the latter is the level of back-up research that doctors and midwives are used to seeing before a new treatment/medicine is given to anyone in their care.

Lack of funding

Besides the scepticism about complementary medicine from much of the traditional medical establishment, another reason why it has few trials backing it is that clinical trials are expensive to run. They are usually funded by wealthy drug companies (when the trial involves the use of their products), the Government, through the Medical Research Council (MRC), and medical charities.

The most recent funding figures show that the MRC did not give any funding to a single project involving complementary therapies in 2001, and that the medical charities only gave 0.05% of their total combined budgets to complementary therapy research.

Acupuncture

Acupuncture is a traditional form of Chinese medicine that has been used in China for at least 2000 years. It only became widely known in the West in the 1970s, when its pain-killing ability led to widespread media coverage.

The therapy is now widely used in the UK, Europe and the USA, especially in the field of pain relief. In the UK it is among the top five most popular and trusted complementary therapies for which people are prepared to pay, and nearly every NHS pain clinic offers it. On the World Health Organisation's list of traditional complementary therapies and the conditions they help, acupuncture is flagged up as being useful for 40 different conditions, including childbirth.

Acupuncturists work on the principle that there are many hundreds of small energy centres called acupoints scattered all over the skin's surface. They are laid out in an orderly way along pathways of invisible energy (*qi* or *chi*) called meridians. Most of these run in a tidy pattern from the upper part of the body and head all the way down to the ends of the fingers, and the *qi* energy is said to travel around the body steadily and constantly, like electricity flowing around a delicate and complex circuitboard.

Some Western scientists have suggested that *qi* is a form of weak electromagnetic energy, and indeed, according to research carried out by the Institute of Electrical and Electronic Engineers, the skin above the meridian pathways does have special electrical properties that the skin in between the pathways does not.

Acupuncture practitioners believe that disease or illness is caused when the smooth flow of *qi* is interrupted or blocked, causing disruption or starvation to the organ or area that it normally supplies. To put this right, an acupuncturist gently inserts the tip of a fine needle or needles a very small way into specific acupoints to unblock and stimulate energy flow to the affected area again.

In a modern variation of the therapy called electro-acupuncture, the needles are wired up to a very gentle, low-dose source of electricity. These are left in place for longer than ordinary needles. This form is especially popular with Western-trained acupuncturists and doctors.

How it works in labour

Acupuncture is believed to help reduce labour pain in two ways:

■ By stimulating the womb to contract strongly and smoothly, so that labour progresses steadily and well.

■ By encouraging the release of the body's own powerful natural pain-killing hormones (endorphins).

There are, in fact, more acupoints for helping labour and delivery go well than there are for relieving pain as such. One reason for this is that in China it was felt that, as long as the labour was going smoothly, women didn't really need pain relief when they had a baby. However, because difficult, delayed or very long labours were seen to be fatal for mothers, their babies, or sometimes both, traditional Chinese physicians did develop sophisticated acupuncture techniques that encourage and re-establish normal labour. This is why there are far more acupoint combinations for speeding up a slow labour, encouraging a non-dilating cervix to open, and helping to turn a breech (bottom-first) birth, than there are for straightforward pain relief.

It also follows that if your labour is going steadily and smoothly, it will generally be much easier for a mother to handle and so will hurt less anyway.

Treating yourself

In order to keep you going until your acupuncturist arrives, ask her to show you some points on your ear or feet that you can stimulate yourself with a match head or the tip of your finger.

How you have it

For relieving labour pain, an acupuncturist will usually insert some fine needles in your ear (and sometimes in your feet), since the pattern of acupoints in your ears mirrors the pattern of points on the rest of your body. The exact positions of the needles will vary a little from practitioner to practitioner.

Between two and five needles are used, and they are left in place for up to half an hour, or removed after only a few minutes if you are in the first stage of labour. These needles don't get in the way of anything, and you can move about freely and even have a bath with them in.

During the early part of labour a very traditional Chinese acupuncturist might also use small bundles of a Chinese herb called *moxa* (mugwort). These are lit to release an aromatic smoke, then held over the body to warm the skin around particular acupoints.

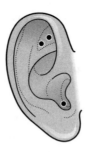

In acupuncture, each area of the body relates to a specific point in the ear. Working with the points (shown left) that relate to areas involved in labour will help to relieve pain

How fast it works

Ear acupuncture (also known as auricular therapy) can start soothing labour pain within a few minutes. For speeding up a slow, non-progressing and exhausting labour (these labours tend to hurt more than swift, easy labours), the effects take 30-60 minutes to be felt and last for 30-60 minutes, so you will probably need more than one treatment during your labour. Some benefits may still be felt 24 hours later.

How effective it is

Practitioners, and mothers who have used acupuncture in labour, say that it reduces the pain by anything from one quarter, which takes a substantial edge off, to two thirds. The amount varies from study to study and from woman to woman.

Much of the clinical research looking at how effective acupuncture is at reducing labour pain or speeding up childbirth and helping it go smoothly has been done in China itself and so the literature is, not unreasonably, in Chinese. However, some of the research has at least a summary in English (see References), and many other studies have been carried out in European countries including Sweden, Austria and Italy, and also in Australia.

Studies at Morrabbin Hospital in Melbourne, Australia, in 1997, found electro-acupuncture made women's contractions stronger and their labour faster. Research at the University Hospital at Malmo, Sweden, in 1998 looked at 180 women in labour, half of whom were given acupuncture for childbirth pain. They found that six out of 10 of the acupuncture mothers gave birth to their babies without needing any other form of pain relief, but fewer than two in 10 of those who didn't have acupuncture managed to do the same. Another study at the University of Vienna Medical School in Austria looked at how 80 women got along when half were given prenatal acupuncture treatment (before they went into labour) and half were not. The treatment group's labours were quicker by two-and-a-half hours on average.

Another Swedish trial published in 1998 looked at the birth records of 3317 women at a single hospital and found that in the two years after the maternity unit started offering acupuncture, there was a drop in the number of women using conventional methods of pain relief. Six out of 10 said the needles gave them good relief from the pain, and eight out of 10 said they wanted to use it the next time they had a baby.

More research in Cyprus looked at 186 women having either their first or second baby, and found that those who had acupuncture had faster labours. And of the women who gave birth within six hours (the average time for the trial), none needed any other sort of pain relief. The

American Journal of Chinese Medicine (1976) also documents cases where acupuncture was used successfully to encourage overdue labours to start.

The people who use it

Acupuncture is the most popular method of natural pain relief in Sweden, where many state hospitals have also carried out extensive research on the subject. This may be partly because the country has some of the most progressive social and health policies in Europe, if not the world, and partly because of the strong movement amongst many Swedish midwives and mothers towards keeping childbirth as natural as possible.

Acupuncture for pain relief in childbirth is slowly gaining acceptance in the UK. And where there are pockets of expertise among midwives, such as in Plymouth and Oxford, it is becoming a popular option for mothers who prefer to use natural rather than drug-based methods of pain relief and labour support.

Ironically, although acupuncture is still quite widely practised in China, many Chinese doctors who are also trained in Western medicine regard it as old-fashioned and not as effective as powerful drugs. So, with a few exceptions, they tend not to use it to help women in labour.

When China opened up to the West in the 1970s, Western countries became interested in traditional Chinese medicine in general and acupuncture and Chinese herbalism in particular. China, to a far greater degree, fell in love with orthodox Western medicine. Up until this point, Chinese surgeons had been routinely performing open-lung surgery, abdominal operations and even brain surgery using electro-acupuncture for many years. Now, operations under acupuncture tend only to be done in major cities, such as Beijing, Nanjing and Shanghai, and often for the benefit of visiting Western VIPs, such as politicians, university professors of medicine and top doctors. It is now more usual for Chinese doctors and obstetricians to use drugs to speed up labour and provide pain relief.

Overdue?

About one in 10 mothers goes up to a week or more past her due date, and faces the possibility of having her baby induced, which can mean a more painful labour and a greater chance of a Caesarean. Acupuncture may be able to get a reluctant labour going naturally within 36 hours. The relevant acupoints for this are on the front of the shin, along the side of the calf and along the side of the hand, from the wrist to the index finger.

Acupuncture – the pros

- It can be an effective way to reduce labour pain. It helps two out of three women who use it, and reduces the level of pain they feel by up to two thirds.
- It's drug-free.
- It may make your labour quicker.
- It may help childbirth go smoothly in other ways.
- There are no major side effects.
- The needles go in only a small way and do not hurt.
- Only a few needles are used, usually in the ear, and so do not get in your way.
- You can remain as mobile as you like.
- You can use other forms of pain relief as well if you need to (possibly not TENS if you are having electro-acupuncture – check with your acupuncturist).
- A couple of visits to an acupuncturist before your due date could get you in good condition for labour and encourage a swift recovery afterwards.

Acupuncture – the cons

- You have to arrange it yourself.
- You need two or three sessions with the practitioner beforehand.
- You usually need to pay. It is only available on the NHS in a very few hospitals, including Plymouth and Oxford, where they have midwife-acupuncturists available. Fees range from £30-£50 for a first consultation, £20-£40 thereafter. You also need to negotiate a fee for the practitioner to attend your labour. Some charge by the hour, which can really mount up if your labour is a long one, so try to arrange a flat fee, which can be anything from £120 upwards.
- You need to have the practitioner in the hospital with you as you cannot do acupuncture yourself. (Your practitioner could show you some helpful acupressure points to press while you are waiting for her to arrive.)
- You have to get permission from the obstetrician in charge of the unit. You may have difficulty in persuading him to agree, so you may need to search

Its use in Caesareans

Beijing Hospital in China still performs 98% of its 1000 Caesareans a year using acupuncture alone. The hospital claims that the mothers choose acupuncture because it works well and has no side effects on the baby.

The way ahead?
Few midwives are trained in acupuncture, yet there could be many thousands. Those who have pioneered and taught acupuncture for midwifery in the UK say that the specific positions for pain relief (not for helping any labour problems) can be taught in a weekend.

around for a more liberal-minded unit.
■ The pain relief you get from acupuncture does vary. Some women find it good, while others find it doesn't work for them at all.
■ Availability. There are few trained midwife acupuncturists, and you may have difficulty finding an acupuncturist with an interest in childbirth who would be willing to be with you in labour.

How you get it
The British Acupuncture Council in London (see Resources) will be able to tell you if there are any professionally trained acupuncturists with an interest in childbirth in your area. Word-of-mouth is another good way of finding a practitioner – ask your midwife, any good complementary health practitioners in your area, or childbirth groups such as the local branch of The National Childbirth Trust.

Aromatherapy
Aromatherapy uses the concentrated scented essences extracted and distilled from many types of plants (trees, flowers, herbs, spices and fruits) to treat mental and physical disorders and promote wellbeing.

There are more than 200 essential (essence) oils, and they are all said to have their own special scent and healing properties. Some, such as Tea Tree, are anti-fungal, others, such as Bergamot, are thought to have an antiseptic action. Many appear to have a calming, uplifting or anti-depressant effect by working on the central nervous system. Only 30 or 40 of the oils are commonly used, including Rose, Cedarwood, Lemon, Rosemary, Lavender, Ginger, Myrrh, Cypress and Juniper Berry. A single oil may have more than one property (type of action).

The principle of aromatherapy is similar to that of herbalism in that aromatherapy draws on the healing power of plants. But instead of using part or all of the plant, it uses just the plant's potent, distinctive-smelling essential oil. Originally seen in Britain as a gentle 'extra something' masseurs and beauticians added to their massage oil to help relax their clients, aromatherapy oils can be more powerful than they sound.

In France, for instance, oils were used by Dr Jean Valnet in the Second World War to treat the appalling wounds of front-line soldiers. As a result, the French take aromatherapy very seriously, and only their qualified doctors can use oils to help diagnose and treat certain types of illness, prescribing them even for internal use.

Over the past 10 years in the UK aromatherapy has quietly been gaining acceptance in several areas of orthodox medicine. It is now used with massage for hospitalised babies, people with cancer and heart disease (some trials have been done on patients following cardiac surgery), people who are HIV positive or living with AIDS, and for those with chronic long-term pain. Some of the small but growing number of new multi-disciplinary GP practices employ an aromatherapist once or twice a week with other complementary practitioners, such as osteopaths, to work alongside the GPs and practice nurses.

How it works in labour

Some interesting studies – one involving more than 8000 women in childbirth – have been done by midwives over the past 10 years at major NHS teaching hospitals in Britain. They suggest that aromatherapy can have a wide variety of benefits for women in labour, including:
- Calming anxiety (midwives and obstetricians agree that this in itself can reduce pain considerably and help labour go more smoothly).
- Soothing labour pain directly. It is thought that the essential oils act on the central nervous system, producing a measure of pain relief by stimulating the release of certain neuro-chemicals, including the natural pain-killing endorphin group. *Lavendula angustifolia* is the best known oil for this.
- Making womb contractions more efficient and powerful. Anything that does this (see Acupuncture, p102) may be

helpful, especially if your labour isn't progressing (you may be having plenty of painful contractions, but your cervix isn't opening, or doing so very slowly). This is more common for first-time mothers. Usually you would be given an intravenous infusion of the artificial version of oxytocin, the naturally occurring hormone that makes your womb contract powerfully. But this can produce contractions that are strong and abrupt and tend to hurt more than naturally occurring ones. In a study of aromatherapy in labour by the midwives at Oxford's John Radcliffe Maternity Hospital in 1990, which involved 585 women, Clary Sage essential oil was successfully used 111 times to help increase the effectiveness of contractions. Another study, in New South Wales, used a mixture of Lavender and Clove (one or two drops of clove added to a warm bath) to stimulate effective contractions.

■ Stimulating the release of different types of neuro-chemicals. Some essences are thought to encourage the output of your body's own sedative, stimulant and relaxing substances. Many also appear to be anti-infective, killing viruses, bacteria and fungal infections, which means they can also be helpful if you have problems after delivery, such as infected stitches.

A quick fix

For an immediate calming effect breathe in the oils from a tissue. The scent stimulates the olfactory centres of the brain – the hippocampus and thalamus – both of which are linked to the hypothalamus, the part of your brain that controls your mood.

How you use it

There are several different ways to use aromatherapy oils.

■ You can breathe them in. Inhale them in a steam infusion by bending your head over a basin of hot water with a few drops in it. Or, more easily done in a labour ward, put a few drops of neat oil onto a tissue or a cool damp face flannel and hold it to your nose. You could also put a few drops on a piece of absorbent card for inhaling, or on your pillow or a beanbag you are using.

When you breathe them in, the essential oil particles come into immediate contact with the roof of your nasal passages. There are tiny sensory cell receptors buried in the protective mucus lining of these passages, and protruding from each one thin hairs called cilia that register and transmit information about the smell you have just inhaled via the olfactory bulb at their root. From here, electro-chemical messages race to the limbic area of the brain, which is associated with your sense of smell.

This is thought to trigger the release of different neuro-chemicals. If you have just inhaled essential oil with sedative properties, such as Cedarwood, aromatherapists feel this encourages your brain to release neuro-chemicals to make you calm and slightly drowsy. Lavender, which can help soothe pain, is thought to trigger the release of hormones from the endorphin group. Endorphins are powerful morphine-like substances that act as natural painkillers. They are produced in impressively large quantities by your body when you go into labour, and are also involved in several other natural methods of pain relief, notably birthing pools, TENS, acupuncture and reflexology.

Most of the oils have more than one type of action. It is not unusual to find one that is said to have analgesic (pain-killing) properties, but which can also induce drowsiness and promote sleep (certain pain-killing drugs, such as morphine and pethidine, have the same effect). Lavender oil is one example.

■ Through massage. Mix the essential oils with a carrier oil and have them massaged into your skin. Massage alone can help reduce pain in labour (p151), but aromatherapists and many midwives say it is far more effective when you use essential oils as well.

Generally, the skin is an efficient barrier. However, very small amounts of essential oil have been shown to seep deep into the pores and hair follicles. Because these structures are rooted in the lowest, living layer of skin, just above the network of blood vessels and nerves, this is thought to be the route by which the oils reach the blood capillaries. Once there they can be transported around your body, and if even tiny amounts reach the nerves, they have direct access to the central nervous system itself.

Massage mix

In the first stage of labour ask your midwife or partner to give you a lower-back massage with a carrier oil containing a blend of Lavender, Melissa, Clary Sage, Jasmine and Rose. Applied for 10-15 minutes every half an hour, this can help relax your muscles and increase your pain tolerance.

During the second stage your partner can do lower-back, foot, face, scalp, neck and shoulder massage with the same oils to help with the pain of contractions.

Essential oil bath

For a pain-relieving and relaxing aromatherapy bath in labour, add five drops of good-quality Lavender oil to a palmful of carrier oil (a plain oil for diluting the essential oils – eg, almond oil) then mix into the warm water.

Some women do not like being touched when they are in labour, and simply want to be left alone, so being massaged or being asked to inhale essential oils might irritate and upset you. Instead, you may find a bath containing essential oils more comforting. Or try putting three drops of Lavender and two of Clary Sage on the neckline of your nightdress or T-shirt, on your pillow or a beanbag, or even on your front hairline if you like the smell.

■ In your bath. Add several drops of essential oil to a bath. Again, small quantities of the oil will be absorbed via your hair follicles and skin pores, and some will be breathed in through the water droplets in the steam. Run a warm bath rather than a hot one, as a hot one could make you dizzy and raise your baby's temperature, which could be harmful to her. Add between six and 10 drops, but check with your midwife first. You need to stay in the water for at least 20 minutes to get the full effect. Lying or sitting in a bath of warm water can be very helpful in itself for soothing pain in labour anyway (p169).

Helpful oils for pain relief

■ Lavender. It must be the *Lavendula angustifolia* variety – check with the supplier as there are several varieties of Lavender and not all are analgesic (pain-soothing). This has a pain-relieving and slightly sedative, calming effect.

■ Clary Sage, which helps the womb contract well and efficiently.

■ Chamomile, which has a calming or uplifting effect, and is possibly pain-relieving, too.

■ Frankincense.

■ Melissa.

■ Rose, though this may be too overpowering a smell for some women, or too expensive.

■ Rosewood.

■ Neroli.

■ Jasmine.

- Bergamot.
- Lemon.
- Mandarin.

How fast it works

If you are inhaling the oils, it takes only two or three minutes to feel the effects, which will last for about 30 minutes to an hour. Massage with essential oils or soaking in a warm bath to which oils have been added starts to take effect after about 10 minutes, and you should feel the full effects after 20 or 30 minutes. However, because massage can continue throughout labour, how long its effects last is difficult to judge.

When you can, and can't, use it

You can use aromatherapy at any stage of your labour, right from the earliest contractions. But always consult a properly trained aromatherapist for advice on which oils to take into the labour room with you, as some can be harmful in pregnancy and childbirth. Do not use oils in a bath or massage if you have a skin condition such as eczema as they could cause further irritation – breathe the oils instead.

How effective it is

Aromatherapy has been successfully used as a method of pain relief in labour at several maternity units in the UK, including those in Ipswich and Southampton. It has also been studied by midwives at Oxford's John Radcliffe Hospital, Hitchinbrooke Hospital in Cambridgeshire and at Oxford Brooks University.

The latter looked at 8085 mothers using aromatherapy and found that Clary Sage and Chamomile were effective at relieving pain, and that Lavender was helpful for soothing anxiety and promoting calm. Another study in 1994, involving nearly 600 women, tried several oils for different things, including pain relief, soothing anxiety, reducing the nausea that some women feel when they are in labour, and increasing the rate or strength of labour

Do you like the smell?
If you don't like the smell of an oil, don't use it. Find an alternative. Many women are especially sensitive to smell when they are giving birth, and no matter how helpful an oil may be physiologically, it is going to do more harm than good if you don't like its scent.

An oil for general use
If you want one general-purpose oil for childbirth, choose *Lavendula angustifolia*. It costs about £6.99 for a 10ml bottle of good quality organic oil.

contractions – 62% per cent of the women said the oils were effective, 12% said they did not help, and the rest were not sure.

According to the aromatherapists' professional umbrella body, the Aromatherapy Organisations Council (and its previous Director of Scientific Research, former pathologist Dr Vivian Lunny, who trains midwives and nurses in the use of essential oils), the pain relief that the oils offer varies. Yet Dr Lunny says that most women would rate their effectiveness at 60-70%. 'This could be even higher,' she says, 'up to 85% if the practitioner is a medical aromatherapist.'

The Oxford Brooks study found that more than half the mothers rated them as helpful. Interestingly, they were not all 'easy' cases – six out of 10 had never had a baby before (first-time mothers are more likely to have more painful labours and complications than mothers who have had a baby before), and one third had had their labours induced (started artificially), which means the contractions tend to be more painful.

Aromatherapy – the pros

- It can be pretty good at relieving labour pain.
Between 50-80% of women who have used it think it is effective.
- It may help your labour go smoothly in other ways, too, perhaps by encouraging effective contractions so your labour progresses steadily.
- There are no recorded negative effects on mother or baby. This is either because there are none or because little research has been carried out into the subject.
- Aromatherapy is compatible with other forms of pain relief, including drugs.
- It is non-invasive.
- It is drug-free.
- Methods of giving aromatherapy are very soothing and nice to have in themselves, especially massage and warm baths.
- It can be helpful after delivery, too.

- It smells good, and so may be a welcome change from the usual smells of a hospital. It may also be agreeable and calming to the other people present at the birth, including your baby, partner and midwife.

Aromatherapy – the cons
- The cost. Aromatherapy in labour is not free on the NHS, unless you happen to be part of a clinical midwifery trial, and some of the oils can be expensive.
- If you want an aromatherapist with you in labour, it may be difficult to find one who has a special interest in childbirth, and who will be willing to come with you to hospital.
- Your hospital may not be happy for you to take an aromatherapist into the labour ward with you, and this might require some tact, persistence and shopping around to resolve.

How to get it
To find a professionally qualified therapist, contact the Aromatherapy Organisations Council (see Resources) and ask which of their members has an interest in childbirth. It is very important to have the help of one who has been properly trained.

Members' fees are a little higher than for therapists who have not done any of the recognised training courses – the latter may only have done a very short course, sometimes no more than a weekend or two. This may be fine if they are offering basic relaxation massages and beauty treatments with essential oils, but they would not be qualified to help you in pregnancy or labour. When you have some names and phone numbers of therapists, speak to them first over the phone and explain to them what you would like.

Aromatherapy for labour pain can be supplied in two ways:
- An aromatherapist comes with you to the labour ward and stays with you until your baby has been born. A qualified therapist would probably charge a flat fee

A specialist birth kit
It's possible to have an aromatherapist make up a kit of suitable oils for you to use in labour (see overleaf).

(negotiate it beforehand) of £100-£250. There would also be a fee of £25-£50 for an initial consultation, which would also include an aromatherapy treatment. Many will charge less if you really need help and have little money so, if fees are a problem, talk this over with them first. Check that they are willing to come with you after-hours or during the night, as babies arrive at unpredictable times, and that they are prepared to spend all night with you if necessary before facing a full quota of clients the next day. It's very important that you like and feel comfortable with the therapist. If you don't, it's best to find someone else, no matter how good this one may be.

■ You take a birth kit containing the most helpful oils with you to the labour ward to use yourself, or keep them handy at home if you're having a home birth. The kit should be made up by a therapist who has an interest in childbirth. If you want to be massaged rather than put the oils in a bath or on a flannel, explain that you would like to show your birth partner (whether it is your husband, boyfriend, friend, mother or sister) the best way to massage you. The consultation will cost £25-£50, and perhaps another few pounds for the oils, though you may not be charged for these.

How to get the oils

There are several good mail-order companies that supply members of the public as well as professional therapists (see Resources). Their oils are usually of much better quality than the budget varieties sold in some high street retail outlets, which tend to smell good but are not very clinically effective.

Oils can be costly. Lavender, Clary Sage and Rosewood are only £5 or £6 for a 10ml bottle (used together they may well provide helpful pain relief), but Melissa is £30-plus for a 10ml bottle, and Rose, Jasmine and Neroli can cost £30-£40 for a mere 2ml. You may need to adjust your mixture of oils to your budget, or buy them by the drop, which is possible if there is an outlet near you.

Be warned

Beware of using cheap oils as they can cause skin rashes. Try to use good quality ones, such as Fragrant Earth or Neal's Yard – or ask an aromatherapist which ones they would suggest. If you want to use the oils when you are pregnant, consult a well-trained practitioner because some of the oils can be harmful in pregnancy. Certain ones have even been implicated in miscarriage.

Autogenic training

Autogenic training (AT) is a deep relaxation therapy based on meditation through six simple mental exercises aimed at relieving stress.

There are said to be more than 3000 published clinical papers giving details of its use in helping with a variety of health problems. It has been used medically in the UK, Europe, Russia, Japan and North America to help with, among other things, high blood pressure, asthma, colitis, irritable bowel syndrome, muscular pain, arthritis, migraine, premenstrual syndrome and bladder disorders. Many psychological problems benefit from AT, too, especially anxiety, insomnia and panic attacks.

AT has also been successfully used, in documented clinical trials, to reduce pain in labour and speed up both the first and second stages.

The method was originally developed in Berlin by German neuro-psychiatrist Dr Johannes Schultz, who noted that hypnosis had a beneficial effect on the health of many of his patients. This led him to devise a set of simple relaxation exercises that could promote similar results without the need for hypnosis. AT works by:
- Helping you to relax deeply, fast.
- Using affirmations to help programme your mind and body for a comfortable, swift and trouble-free labour. (Affirmations are positive, 'can-do' instructions that you give to yourself when you are at your most relaxed and receptive.)

You are taught the technique over an eight-week period, either in a group or one-to-one. You need to start learning AT reasonably early in your pregnancy, preferably no later than your sixth month. While you are learning you need to practise the routine twice a day (say, in the morning when you get up, and in the evening before you go to bed). When you have completed the course, try to practise every day or, at the very least, two or three times a week, to keep your hand in. The more you practise, the better it will work for you when you need it.

How you use it

You can use AT in several ways to help make your labour quicker and less painful:

■ By doing the full AT routine when your labour is only just beginning (the latent phase) then adding in an affirmation at the end to the effect that your labour will be smooth, rapid and pain-free.

'I practised the routine daily in the run-up to labour. I think it helped – at least it gave me something else to focus on, besides my contractions'

■ By going through the mental exercise routine in early labour once, twice or three times to achieve and remain in a state of deep calm and relaxation (at this point your contractions may only be coming every 20-30 minutes or so). Or go through the routine at any point when your contractions are far enough apart for you to fit it in between them.

■ By adapting the mental exercises and the passive concentration they produce to coincide with the rhythm of your labour pains, so that the deepest and most effective part of each exercise ('It breathes me', see 5-Step AT routine for pregnant women, opposite) coincides with the peak of each contraction. This is thought to be the most effective way to use AT, although it is also the most complicated.

There are five basic exercises you follow to achieve pain relief in childbirth (the usual routine has six, but there is one that pregnant women are advised not to do because it may increase the blood supply to their abdomen too much). At the end of each one there is a period of peaceful meditation that you can use purely for relaxation or as an opportunity to do an affirmation.

An affirmation is an instruction to the mind, such as 'My labour will be comfortable and pain-free', 'My labour will go easily and naturally' or if you are having, say, sleep problems, 'I will allow myself to fall asleep easily and quickly tonight'. Affirmations are best slipped in when you have meditated peacefully for a little while because your mind will be more receptive to them.

5-Step AT routine for pregnant women

The phrase in brackets is repeated three times, with some calm quiet time to experience and enjoy the sensation of relaxation/warmth, coolness or whatever you are initiating in between:

1. Heaviness: concentrate on feeling a heavy relaxation in your arms, legs, shoulders and neck ('My arms and legs are heavy').

2. Warmth: concentrate on feeling warmth in your arms and legs ('My arms and legs are heavy and warm').

3. Heart: concentrate on your own heartbeat ('My heartbeat is calm and regular'). You may need to leave this one out as it can cause discomfort for pregnant women, whose circulatory system is already working far harder than usual due to a 50% increase in the amount of blood in their body. Discuss this with your AT instructor.

4. Breath: become aware of your breathing ('It breathes me' – this sounds odd but what it means is that your breathing mechanism is working independently on your behalf. Your body is literally breathing for you, or 'breathing you').

5. Cool forehead: concentrate on a feeling of coolness across your forehead ('My forehead is cool and clear'). And finally, as a way of allowing some quiet, calm meditation time, repeat 'I am at peace'.

How fast it works

Once you have completed the AT course and learned to relax deeply and rapidly (people can often do this after just two classes and two weeks' practice), the intense relaxation effects can start kicking in as soon as you go into the routine, with the full effect coming into force as soon as you have finished the exercises.

If you are doing the full routine from one to three times (the usual way of producing relaxation in ordinary circumstances), it would take between about eight and 25 minutes to complete. The pain-relieving effect can last for as long as it is needed.

A quick routine
Doing all five exercises once takes 8-10 minutes, and even this will have a powerful relaxing effect. Doing the complete routine the recommended three times has the maximum effect.

119

When you can use it

You can use AT in any stage of labour. It can also be helpful after the birth for general relaxation and in helping to deal with the fourth-day blues that most women experience to some degree.

AT offers another major bonus for new parents, too, as it can be used to alleviate the sleep problems that most have for many months after their baby is born. AT can be used to make sure you can go to sleep in the first place then go back to sleep fast after your baby has woken you (something many new mothers cannot do), and that if your sleep's only in two-hour snatches, it is deep and refreshing.

There are no times when you can't use AT in childbirth, and it is compatible with other methods of pain relief.

How effective it is

The studies looking at women using AT in childbirth found that:
- About two thirds of the mothers said the pain relief it gave them was 'good' or 'very good'.
- AT makes labours shorter by an average of one third. This applied equally to mothers having their first baby (first-baby labours usually take longer) and to those who had already had a baby.

Much of the research supporting AT has been carried out by Professor Prill of Wurzburg University's Department of Obstetrics, who has done several studies on AT for women in labour, one of which involved more than 1000 mothers. A good deal of the relaxation training done with pregnant women today is based on his work. Several studies carried out in Kyoto in Japan, in China, and also in Italy, at the University of Verona's Institute of Obstetrics & Gynaecology and at the University of Pisa's Department of Obstetrics & Gynaecology, back him up (see References).

One explanation of how AT might help was found by the Pisa group of obstetricians, who noticed that women's levels of endorphins, the body's powerful natural pain-killing hormones, increased remarkably when they learned and practised AT in the last part of their pregnancy and used it in their labours.

Autogenic training – the pros
- Two out of three women who have used it said the pain relief it gives is 'good' or 'very good'.
- It usually shortens labour by one third.
- It works very fast and provides almost instantaneous calmness and relaxation as you go into the relaxation routine.
- It is under your own control.
- There are no side effects for mother or baby.
- It is drug-free.
- It is helpful for other difficulties after the birth.
- Once learned, it is an easy and effective method of reducing stress in all kinds of circumstances.

Autogenic training – the cons
- It takes practice, and it can be difficult finding the time for this if you have other children at home needing your attention, are still working while pregnant, or both.
- It can be time-consuming going to eight weekly training sessions, especially if you are going to weekly antenatal classes as well.
- It costs money to take an AT training course (£100-£200 or so for a group course, and more for individual tuition).
- It does not offer total pain relief as, say, an epidural might.
- It does not work for everybody.

How you get it
You need to find a properly trained instructor to teach you how to do AT. There are more than 100 qualified teachers countrywide. To find one in your area, contact the British Society for Autogenic Training (see Resources). A teacher will show you one exercise per week and help you

Quick route to relaxation
You can learn AT more quickly, and get major results from it faster, than you can with other forms of relaxation, such as those taught in ordinary antenatal and Active Birth classes, yoga and Transcendental Meditation.

deal with any temporary difficulties that may arise from the training.

Some hospitals, including the Royal London Homeopathic Hospital, have AT therapists on staff offering training and treatment on the NHS. However, these are generally reserved for medical and surgical cases. Some are attached to cardiac units, for example, to help people who have had life-threatening heart problems.

It is vital to have an AT teacher who is also properly qualified in one of the caring professions, perhaps as a nurse, doctor, counsellor or psychologist. The technique can sometimes release long-buried psychological and physical problems that you may need temporary help to deal with. For the same reason, it's not a good idea to use a book to teach yourself AT. It will give you the information but not the skilled support and back-up.

Breathing and relaxation

Tension, anxiety and fear are key players in your perception of pain. And that's not because pain is all in the mind, but because there are solid physiological reasons why these factors can, and do, increase the pain you feel.

Anxiety triggers a fall in your body's level of natural pain-soothing hormones called endorphins, while at the same time increasing its output of adrenaline-like hormones called catecholamines. The latter have an important role in labour but you don't want them too early on – their job is to encourage your womb to make those powerful expulsive contractions that push your baby out. If you produce them too early they interfere with the first-stage contractions that help make your womb smaller and open up your cervix. Catecholamines are also pain transmitters in their own right.

Fast work
Relaxation, breathing and visualisation, used separately or together, can work fast, often within just a few minutes.

Fear, tension and pain all feed off each other and can create a vicious circle that is difficult to break. The rationale for education about childbirth is to help women understand, and therefore not be afraid of, what is happening. Many natural pain-relief methods for labour, such as breathing, visualisation, massage, self-hypnosis and autogenic training, also work by helping to remove any fear or tension, thereby reducing and relieving pain.

This is why relaxation is one of the two main foundation stones of most forms of 'mind control' pain relief you can do for yourself (and slow deep steady breathing is vital because it's one of the fastest ways to relax yourself). Being given full information about what will happen during childbirth is the other.

> 'I think there is a difference between pain relief (getting rid of it or reducing it) and coping with the pain, though physically it stays at the same level. Relaxation and breathing is a good way of coping, without actually relieving it'

Any relaxation technique can be adapted to use in childbirth, including yoga, self-hypnosis, autogenic training and different types of meditation. However, The National Childbirth Trust and the Active Birth movement both teach a straightforward form of breathing control and relaxation in their classes especially for use during labour (both organisations run relaxation and preparation-for-childbirth classes countrywide – see Resources).

The big 1990 National Birthday Trust Survey on pain relief in labour in the UK found that about one third of women use relaxation and breathing in their labours (the figure is probably higher now). However, only 3.8% of midwives recorded that their patients used it. This may be because the mothers didn't mention it, the midwives didn't notice (breathing and relaxation is usually a fairly quiet, low-key activity), or because the only pain relief methods usually recorded by hospitals are the ones they provide in the form of drugs.

From an effectiveness point of view, nine out of 10 women said breathing and relaxation was either 'good' or 'very good'.

Relaxation as pain relief

Relaxation used as a form of pain relief is deep relaxation. This is not what many people think of as relaxation –

Relaxation really works

The more relaxed and calm you can be, the less your labour and birth are likely to hurt. Relaxation, breathing for labour, autogenic training, self-hypnosis, water, aromatherapy, reflexology, visualisation and homeopathy can all help to relax and calm you.

they're more likely to think of it as sitting down with their feet up, watching TV and drinking tea. But while it may look as though you're not doing much sitting in front of that TV, your mind is still working and your body may still be tense. And simply lying down for a rest isn't enough either – though your body might not technically be doing anything, it can still be tense in places, and your mind may be refusing to switch off.

Deep relaxation is a different activity altogether because it involves both your body and mind. It could be described as a systematically and deliberately induced state of mental calm, combined with looseness and ease in the body and deep regular breathing.

Of all the body's involuntary physical processes (the ones that carry on happening without you consciously thinking about them), breathing is the easiest one to bring under your control. It encourages relaxation because just by breathing slowly and deeply you can alter other aspects of your nervous system, too, and gain control over your general levels of tension.

When you are feeling anxious your breathing is more rapid and shallow. Many naturally nervous people say that most of the time they feel they are only breathing 'halfway down', and if you are in pain your breathing will be like that. But if you can deepen and slow it you will have a direct effect on the other physical processes of your body, such as your heart rate and blood pressure, and it will also encourage true deep relaxation.

Several forms of yoga and meditation use slow deep breathing to reach altered mental states. In deep meditation an individual might breathe only about three or four times a minute. Those who have trained in the discipline for many years may only breathe once or twice a minute.

How you use it in labour

In the past, breathing for childbirth meant practising different styles of breathing at different points in the contraction – deep breathing at the beginning and middle, then shallow panting at the end. However, this was not always helpful as some women found this too complicated, and some started their shallow breathing too soon. Steady, deep, strong breathing throughout is far easier and it still works.

Practise breathing and relaxation as often as possible, because the more you do it, the easier you will find it and the better it will work for you. Try to set aside 15 or 20 minutes a day that are solely yours. Make sure you are not going to be disturbed – ask your partner to keep any children you may already have out of earshot, and unplug the phone if you might be able to hear it when it rings. Before you start the breathing and relaxation, have a warm, soothing bath or play a favourite piece of calming music for a few minutes to help settle you. Mentally, put any outstanding business and all your worries in a large box or lidded basket, then 'see' yourself shutting it firmly with a lock and key, so it can be opened later and its contents dealt with when your relaxation has finished.

> 'It's something that helps, and you can do it yourself – you don't have to ask the midwife to give it to you. This makes all the difference'

Breathing for labour

The more you practise breathing and relaxation, the faster you will be able to slip into it, the more deeply you will be able to relax, and the more it will help you in labour. Try the following simple exercises.

Exercise 1: Just breathing

The idea of practising breathing may sound silly because we breathe all the time. But breathing, and being aware of how you are doing it, are two different things.

Breathing in an ordinary way, without thinking about it, keeps you alive. But being aware of your breath enables you to control it. When you can do that – and you may find you can do so very quickly – it can help you cope with any pain you feel.

1. First, get really comfortable. Wriggle about a bit until you are.

2. Rest your feet on the floor, hands loosely on your lap or thighs, and your back supported in an upright chair. Or lie back in a comfortable armchair. Some women find sitting on the floor with their knees bent and legs crossed very comfortable, perhaps with their back supported by a wall.

3. Close your eyes. Or if you prefer, leave them open but do not focus on a particular spot – try to develop a blank unfocused stare instead.

4. Just breathe out slowly. This out-breath part of your breathing cycle is the relaxing part – notice how your body starts to let go and loosen as you do it. This is the part you will be concentrating on to release tension and help you cope with the pain.

Exercise 2: Relaxing as you breathe

Tensing up and holding your breath is a common, instinctive reaction to something hurting. Many women do this during labour, and it can mean they then experience more pain. The following can help you overcome this natural reaction (it may sound complicated, but all you are really doing is tensing each bit of your body in turn as you breathe in, and releasing it as you breathe out):

1. Start by breathing as slowly, evenly and deeply as you can. Concentrate on doing this for a while, perhaps five minutes. Let it settle into an easy rhythm.

2. Relax your body, starting with your forehead. Breathe in and frown as you do so, then breathe out, letting the frown go smooth again.

3. Now it's time for your face. Breathe in and scrunch it up, then breathe out and relax it again, letting your lower jaw drop a little so your lips part slightly. Make sure your tongue isn't clamped against the roof of your mouth, or its tip pushing hard against your front teeth. Feel your face becoming softer and smoother.

4. Next come the shoulders. Breathe in and shrug them up to your ears, at the same time flexing your arms at the elbow and clenching your fists. Breathe out, letting your shoulders drop back down, relaxing your arms

Quick way to relax
The quickest way to relax deeply is also the easiest and simplest – just change the way you breathe.

and stretching/flexing your fingers and wrists. Do this
part of the exercise two or three times if you wish – the
shoulders, hands and neck are usually the tensest parts
of the body.
5. Breathe in and make your neck as long as you can,
then out again, allowing it to sink gently back to its
original position.
6. Now for your back.
Breathe in and arch
gently to stretch the
back, then breathe out
and let it go. Breathe in
again, pulling your shoulder blades in together,
stretching your upper back, and then let that go.

> 'I blew the pains away as hard as I could each time they came. It was not pain relief as such, but I found that if I did this I could cope OK'

7. Breathe in and tighten up your abdominal muscles.
Notice what this does to your breathing. Let that breath
out again and relax the abdominals.
8. Breathe in and tighten your bottom and pelvic floor.
If you are not sure which muscles are the ones in your
pelvic floor, they are the ones you would use if you
needed to simultaneously stop a bowel movement and
hold in a very full bladder. As you breathe out, let those
muscles relax, imagining tension flowing out of you as
you do so.
9. Breathe in and tighten your thigh muscles, then relax
them as you breathe out. Do the same with your calf
muscles.
10. Breathe in as you flex your feet upwards towards
the ceiling from your ankles, then breathe out and relax
them again.
11. Breathe in, curling your toes tightly. Breathe out and
let go. Now just breathe in and out, slowly and deeply for
a while, feeling all the tension flow out of your body each
time you exhale, and sinking gently into a deeper state
of relaxation.

It may be difficult to do this exercise while reading the
instructions. If so, ask a friend to read them in a calm,
quiet voice as you follow them, or record them onto tape
for yourself.

Blow away the pain
If breathing-for-labour techniques sound all very well but possibly a bit much when you're in full-throttle labour, try the easy way. Just blow, rather than simply release, each breath, as if you were blowing the pain away.

Mental relaxation and visualisation

Once your body is relaxed, it is time to still your mind. Sometimes when your body relaxes your mind goes into overdrive, imagining detailed conversations with people you know, having creative ideas relating to work, making shopping lists – doing anything other than allowing you to switch it off for a while. However, you can often soothe, still and focus your mind by visualisation, which means imagining something so clearly that you can see it in your mind's eye.

Images that can be helpful and relaxing include a peaceful scene in the country, a deserted beach you once went to, a place under a tree by a river, and a favourite armchair by the fire – in short, anywhere you feel secure and happy. Try to recreate all the details of how it looks, as if you are painting a picture in your mind, and hold it there. Soon you will be concentrating on that rather than on what's going on around you (see also hypnotherapy, p143). It is far easier to do this when your body is relaxed and your breathing deep than when you are in your usual state of consciousness.

When you feel rested and ready, wake yourself up gradually. Wriggle your fingers and toes, stretch, yawn, open your eyes, wait a few moments, then get up slowly. Do not try to get up immediately as your blood pressure can drop measurably during deep relaxation and you could feel dizzy or faint.

Visualisation in labour

In 17th-century France a woman in labour often had a lighted candle and a particular type of rose, the Rose of Jericho, in holy water placed next to her. The heat of the burning candle made the rose's petals open out gradually, mirroring the way her body was slowly opening to let her baby out. This particular rose also had a special religious meaning as it was said to have blossomed for the first time at the birth of Christ, closed when he was crucified, and then opened again on the day he rose from the dead (its other name is the Resurrection Flower).

While French women 300 years ago concentrated on a real rose opening and imagined their bodies doing the same, women in relaxation-for-childbirth classes today are often taught to visualise their cervix opening like a flower unfolding or ripening like a soft fruit. As your cervix opens, visualise your baby moving steadily down your vagina, which you could see as soft and stretchy.

When to use these techniques

You can use relaxation, breathing and visualisation techniques at any time, and they can be used with all forms of pain-relieving drugs. Especially helpful times include:

■ When your contractions are becoming regular and show a pattern, to help ground yourself at the beginning of your labour. Recent research with mothers at the Milton Hershey Medical Centre in Pennsylvania found that if you start the special patterned breathing too early on (perhaps when your contractions have only just begun, are still irregular and a long way apart), it can really tire you out.

■ When your contractions start to feel painful.

■ At any time during the first stage. Imagining your cervix opening steadily and gently can be very helpful, especially if you become 'stuck' at a certain point.

■ During transition. If you try to shut out everything else for a while you can imagine yourself in a calm place where only you are allowed to set foot. When the contractions are becoming very frequent and intense, and if you are feeling you're losing your ability to cope with them, try visualising them as waves and see yourself riding with them.

■ As you are pushing your baby out. Visualise your birth canal as soft and stretchy.

Breathing in labour itself

If your contractions become too strong and you forget to breathe steadily and deeply, don't worry. Just breathe the best way you can during them, and use relaxation and deep breathing in the intervals in between contractions

What is visualisation?
Visualisation is seeing in your mind's eye a picture of something that is not able to be seen in reality at that moment. It harnesses the enormous power of your mind and imagination, and is an easy technique to learn.

Surf your contractions

Another way to use visualisation in labour is to imagine pain itself in a different way – perhaps seeing the contractions as huge, warm, rolling waves that you can effortlessly surf, float or ride over, flowing onto a peaceful empty beach.

instead. Ask your partner to breath in a slow, deep steady rhythm to help you. Not noisily, right in your ear, but near to you, perhaps as you lean into him while he is holding or supporting you. Being held by someone who is breathing calmly and deeply can be very soothing in its own right as well as helping you to re-establish your own breathing pattern.

Having a partner alongside, breathing in the right rhythm, is particularly important for women who have had pethidine, as the drug can occasionally cause them to become so relaxed that they forget to breathe at all.

Breathing and relaxation – the pros

- It can offer good pain relief.
- It works fast.
- It is under your own control.
- There are no side effects for mother or baby.
- You can use it at any point during labour, and it's useful afterwards, too.
- Its effects last throughout labour and can leave you feeling calmer afterwards, even when you have stopped using the technique.
- There are no circumstances under which it would not be helpful.
- You can combine it with all other forms of pain relief if required.
- It's drug-free.

Breathing and relaxation – the cons

- It does not offer total pain relief.
- It does not work well for all women, as some find relaxation techniques more difficult than others.
- It takes time and practice to learn. You would, for best results, need at least a month of antenatal classes and home practice to become sufficiently used to doing it for it to be of real help during labour.
- You need to pay for classes to help you learn the technique. Costs vary depending on where you live. Hospital antenatal classes will probably tell you about

the technique, but will not have much time to spend on showing you how to do it, perhaps just a single lesson to give you the basic idea.

Doulas (people as pain relief)

A doula is a sympathetic, informed and experienced lay person (a non-medical person), who stays with you and supports you during labour. Ideally, she would be a calm, older mother or grandmother figure who has had good experiences of giving birth herself, and some sound basic education about the process of childbirth.

A doula remains with you throughout your labour and birth, giving you practical non-medical help and back-up. This might include offering back, shoulder and head massages, providing you with light snacks and drinks, helping you change and hold positions such as squatting, helping you in and out of a bath, protecting your privacy, giving encouragement – or simply just being a comforting, reassuring presence. 'The most effective doula I know does not touch women in labour,' says Dr Michel Odent, water birth pioneer and supporter of the development of the doula movement in Britain. 'She is just always not far away (she herself has had four babies, including three home births).'

Your doula may help relieve pain because she gives you confidence, helps keep you calmer and makes it easier for you to relax. All these things can have a major effect on the amount of pain you feel in labour and on how smoothly it goes. A smoother, more straightforward childbirth hurts far less than a difficult one.

When you can have one

You can benefit from doula support at any time during your labour. However, ideally it should be someone you and your partner have been able to get to know while you were pregnant, and who then stays with you all through your labour. Many doulas will also visit you at home after the birth to help with breastfeeding and early baby and

After your baby's birth
Deep relaxation and slow breathing are also useful for helping you get to sleep, or back to sleep, both in the noisy maternity ward and when you bring your baby home.

home care, doing the sort of things your own mother or a sister would do. They may visit for anything from a few days afterwards to a few months.

How effective it is

Research in Texas in the 1970s, in Guatemala in 1991, in Botswana in 1998, and in Ohio in 1999 has shown that having a doula with you throughout childbirth can:
- Shorten your labour.
- Result in you needing less pain relief and reduce the likelihood of you needing an epidural by more than 80%.
- Reduce the likelihood of you needing a Caesarean by 50%, and make it less likely that your baby will need to be delivered using forceps or ventouse.

The studies carried out in Texas, Guatemala and Ohio also showed that the women having this one-to-one practical and emotional support had fewer babies that needed special care. However, another study, in California, didn't find that doulas made any difference. Interestingly, the women who took part in the Californian study all had their male partners with them as well throughout labour, whereas the women from the other studies did not. This has led some birth experts to wonder whether the doula effect works best if the doula and the woman in labour are alone, with the father waiting elsewhere until the baby has been born.

Research carried out in 1990 supports this thinking. It suggests first-time dads offer less practical support than a doula does. The researchers found that doulas touched the mother 95% of the time (holding her, rubbing her back, stroking her), but the men touched their partners less that 20% of the time, and spent less time in the labour room, too. However, new studies in Hong Kong show that having your partner with you in labour may ensure you are in less pain.

Doulas – the pros
- They may reduce the likelihood of you having a Caesarean or assisted delivery with forceps or ventouse,

and of your baby needing special care after the birth.
■ They may considerably reduce your need for ordinary pain relief.
■ They help you feel more relaxed, calm and confident.
■ It's a drug-free method.
■ Doulas can be a great help in supporting you when you first go home with your baby, too. In some countries, including the UK, doulas can also help with the housework, cooking and care of other young children in the first few weeks or months, and will also help you establish breastfeeding.

Doulas – the cons
■ You will need the maternity unit's permission to have a doula with you in hospital.
■ You have to find and arrange a doula yourself.
■ You must pay them for their time.
■ You need to spend time getting to know your doula before your labour – at least a couple of home visits.
■ Results seem to be better when it's just the doula and the mother in the labour room, with checks and monitoring from a midwife or obstetrician as necessary. So you may need to choose between having your doula or your partner with you for much of the time.

How you get one
The National Childbirth Trust, local Active Birth Centre teachers and La Leche League are likely to know of doulas in your area (for more organisations and for commercial maternity nurse and doula agencies, see Resources). Try to contact more than one in your area if possible. Speak to them over the phone and arrange to meet up for a chat. It's essential that you like your doula. If you don't, and no matter how experienced she is, it will be better for you to find another one.

Costs vary depending on where you live, but expect to pay about £200-£250 for attending your labour and birth, then £7-£10 per hour when at home afterwards, usually for a minimum of half a day at a time. Mothers usually have doulas helping them at home for anything from a week to three months, but you will be able to request just one follow-up visit if finances are a problem or that's all you'd like.

Homeopathy

The word homeopathy comes from an Ancient Greek phrase meaning 'similar suffering', and it's based on the principle that like will cure like. To help someone who is unwell or in pain, a homeopath will prescribe minute, safe doses of the things that can, in larger quantities, produce the very symptoms they are trying to cure. All homeopathic remedies work by gently stimulating the body's own defence systems so that it can heal itself. Homeopaths work according to three principles:

■ The ancient Law of Similars, which states that whatever substance causes harm can also cure it. Coffea, the homeopathic preparation derived from coffee, is one example. Several cups of coffee late at night can stimulate your nervous system and give you the jitters, with insomnia to boot. But when the derivative is given in minute homeopathic preparations it has the opposite effect, soothing the nerves and promoting sleep.

■ The Minimum Dose, which means that only the tiniest amount is needed as a stimulus to cause a reaction. This is why homeopathic medicines are diluted and shaken up to tens of thousands of times. They're so diluted, in fact, that conventional methods of analysis can find no trace of the original substance. Homeopaths and other therapists and healers who work with energy medicine (see References) say no matter how much you dilute a substance it will leave behind a faint 'energy echo' of itself. It is this echo that does the work in homeopathic medicines. The weaker the homeopathic remedy you give someone, the weaker the energy echo, yet the more powerful its effect.

This is not easy for most conventionally trained

doctors to understand, because orthodox medicine works on the opposite principle. That is, the bigger the dose of drugs you give, the more effective they'll be.
■ The Single Remedy, which means that it's best to use only one type of remedy at a time, not a mixture.

How it works in labour

Homeopathic remedies are not only prescribed on the basis of a person's physical symptoms, but also on how that person is feeling emotionally.

If you are in labour, a homeopath will choose a remedy according to what sort of pains you are having and how you are feeling in yourself. Different mothers express different emotions in childbirth – no two are exactly alike. So a mother who has got a heavy, dull backache and who feels irritable and frightened, will be given a different remedy from a mother who is experiencing sharp stabbing pains across her lower tummy, but who feels distant and calm. And because you will be feeling and experiencing a variety of things throughout your labour, you will probably need different remedies at different times.

While homeopathy does not eliminate pain in labour in the way that an epidural can, practitioners say that it will:
■ Subtly stimulate your own physiological system so it functions well and strongly, perhaps by strengthening your womb contractions so that your cervix opens smoothly and steadily.
■ Help you cope well and take labour in your stride.
■ Calm, soothe and relax you, which in itself will reduce the amount of pain you are feeling.

Remedies for labour

Some of the homeopathic remedies that are used most often in labour include:
■ Arnica, to help reduce bruising, swelling and trauma. This is perhaps the best known and most widely used of all homeopathic remedies in childbirth.
■ Caulophyllum, if you are getting needle-like pains in

your cervix, leaving you fretful and shivering.

- Belladonna, if your contractions are very violent and powerful.
- Bellis perennis, for any deep abdominal surgery, including a Caesarean.
- Cimicifuga, if you have pains that shoot right across the front of your abdomen or go down your hips on either side. These may be irregular and they may make you shiver and shake.
- Coffea, if your pains are very strong and painful. This is often helpful for women who are usually highly active and are experiencing excessively painful contractions.
- Gelsemium, for violent contractions that don't seem to be dilating your cervix, which remains rigid.
- Kali carb, for when all the pain seems to be in your lower back, especially if the only thing that helps is someone rubbing very hard on the area.

And, for other forms of discomfort and distress:
- Nux vomica, if you are continually wanting to pass water and have a strong urge to push before it is time to do so. Also for cramping and spasmodic contractions, especially if you are very irritable.

How you have it

Homeopathic remedies are taken in the following ways:
- Lactose (sugar) tablets, each about half the size of a Haliborange vitamin C pill.
- Powders.
- Granules, the size of tiny ball-bearings.

All these can be dissolved on the tongue or mixed with water that you then take via a dropper. It is much easier for women in labour to swallow liquid than tiny pills, especially if the remedies need to be taken every five minutes. If you have only pills, ask your partner or midwife to crush them with a plastic spoon and mix them with water for you.

All remedies come in different potencies. Potency 6 is the lowest, and it's this one that's usually available from chemists and health shops. Potency 30, which is higher, is available from some specialist suppliers (see Resources). High potencies – 200 and above – are useful if a situation is urgent, but these are best prescribed by a trained homeopath.

How fast it works

If the correct remedy is given in the right dose you will get relief within five to 30 minutes. In an acute situation, such as labour, you can take a remedy every five, 10 or 15 minutes as required. When it starts to make an improvement the dose is decreased, and when the improvement is established you can stop taking it. If there is no improvement after two or three doses, the remedy is the wrong one.

The effect of homeopathic remedies lasts for varying amounts of time, depending on which potency is used and how acute the situation is. If the potency is 200, you may only need to take one dose. If the potency is 6, you may need to take doses every 10 to 30 minutes. Should the effect wear off, you can always have more – homeopathic treatments are not rationed or in fixed doses, as drug pain relief is.

When you can have it

It is safe to take homeopathic remedies during any stage of your pregnancy and labour and after the birth. There are no known circumstances in which it would be inadvisable or dangerous to use homeopathy. It is not possible to overdose on remedies, and if the wrong remedy has been given it will simply have no effect at all.

It's also worth knowing that some of the remedies can be useful for your partner, too, if he is getting worried or upset. Apart from anything else, his distress may also upset you and distract you from what you are doing. Aconite, for fear or worry, is a useful one here. Homeopathy is also safe to give to newborn babies.

How effective it is

It sounds as though something so subtle would be of little use in a powerful and often painful process such as

Avoiding the drip
Caulophyllum may help if you're having painful contractions that aren't making your cervix dilate as it should. If this happens, your midwife may suggest giving you an intravenous drip containing artificial oxytocin to help things along. Although a drip can be effective, the contractions it produces tend to hurt more, so it's a good idea to avoid this if you can. If the homeopathy does not help, you can always have the drip afterwards.

childbirth, but this therapy is said to work extremely well in acute situations. It has been known to stop haemorrhages and has been successfully used immediately after major accidents.

Practitioners claim that many women don't need conventional pain relief at all when their labours are supported homeopathically. Midwives and doctors trained in homeopathy have also given accounts of breech babies turning into the right position for delivery, and Caesareans being avoided because of these remedies (see References).

There are many research studies about the use of homeopathy in labour, but none that we could find looks specifically at pain relief as such. So it's not possible to say that homeopathy will reduce labour pain by, say, one third, as acupuncture or self-hypnosis often will. However, there are several research studies that suggest homeopathy is effective at relieving other types of severe pain, from tooth extraction to migraine.

As to its effectiveness in helping other aspects of labour go smoothly, most of the research looks good. Many of the available clinical studies cover how homeopathic remedies can solve specific problems (some of them quite serious, such as haemorrhaging after childbirth) or how they help labour to progress smoothly and swiftly. In one small study in 1990, the department of Obstetrics and Gynaecology at the University of Milan gave 22 first-time mothers Caulophyllum and compared their progress with 34 other women in labour who weren't given anything. The homeopathically treated women had labours that were about 90 minutes shorter than the other women's.

Another study in the same year at the Kiev Medical Institute looked at 206 women at risk of labour problems associated with the way their womb worked. Some were given conventional medical treatments, such as artificial oestrogenic hormones, while the others received homeopathic treatments, including Caulophyllum and Pulsatilla. Both groups underwent careful monitoring, including scans, fetal heart monitoring and clinical examinations. The homeopathic treatments were found to be as effective as the drugs in treating the problems.

Similar results were found after an open study at Bruhl's Marienhospital, Germany, in 1999. The study compared homeopathic remedies with a conventional anti-spasmodic drug called Buscopan to see which was best at treating women whose cervixes were not opening or who were in excessive pain while they did so. Both treatments were equally effective.

Homeopaths suggest women take Arnica Montana in labour to help reduce bruising and bleeding. In 1990 the Department of Obstetrics & Gynaecology at the University of Witwatersrand, Johannesburg, ran a trial involving 159 women who had had an episiotomy or perineal tear. The findings confirmed the remedy's effectiveness.

In 1995 Professor Parimel Banerji, President of the International Society of Advanced Homeopathy, and Dr Santwana Mukherjee, Research Director of the Institute of Advanced Homeopathy in India, reported to a major international homeopathy congress in New Delhi about their involvement in treating more than 2000 women having home births in the Calcutta area. In every case they used only homeopathy. Their paper claims that although there were labour complications in 15% of cases, 'these were brought under control easily only by using exclusively our homeopathic medicines'.

An aid to coping
Homeopathy does not reduce pain in the same way that a drug or acupuncture does – it works by making labour more efficient and helping you to cope better emotionally.

Homeopathy – the pros
■ It can be very effective in helping women cope with labour, both emotionally and physically.
■ It can help labour go smoothly.
■ Some studies suggest it can correct labour problems.
■ It may shorten labour.
■ It's gentle and non-invasive.
■ There are no recorded side effects for mother or baby.
■ It's widely available, though you have to arrange it yourself.
■ The medication itself is inexpensive if you are simply taking a homeopath's advice on general remedies for a birth kit.

- It can be used throughout pregnancy and labour, and can also help with postnatal problems, such as sore episiotomy sites and breastfeeding difficulties.
- It can work quickly.
- It can be repeated as necessary.
- The medical profession seems to find homeopathy one of the most acceptable forms of complementary medicine, as there are five NHS homeopathic hospitals in Britain and many good clinical trials documenting the therapy's use in different areas of medicine. This may be helpful if you find yourself having to persuade your maternity unit to allow you to have a homeopath with you in labour.

Homeopathy – the cons

- It does not offer pain relief as such. However, by calming you, helping your body to work as it needs to, and encouraging the birth to go smoothly, you will naturally feel less pain, possibly a lot less.
- It does not work for everyone.
- The effectiveness of homeopathy is reduced if other forms of pain relief are given, too, especially if they are powerful pain-killing drugs or strong complementary therapies, such as aromatherapy, because they sledgehammer its gentle effects.
- It can be expensive if you want a homeopath with you during your labour.
- Although homeopathy is accepted by many doctors as a legitimate therapy – and many are trained in it – not all hospitals, nor all consultants, are happy to let you have a homeopath with you in the labour ward (p99).

How you get it

A trained practitioner can help you prepare a basic birth kit of potentially useful remedies for pregnancy, labour and recovery (ask for written instructions on how to use it). But because it's best to have remedies customised for you individually, it's a good idea to have a thorough consultation with a homeopath a couple of months before

Calming fears
Homeopathy can be very helpful for women who feel frightened or panicky during their labour. Two of the best remedies are Aconite 30 for shock or fear, and Calc carb 6 or 30 for protection and stability if you feel especially vulnerable or if you feel things around you are changing too fast.

your baby is due. (If you can't afford a homeopath's fees, ask for advice at a specialist homeopathic pharmacy – see Resources.)

During the consultation you will not only be asked about your medical history but also about your personality and temperament, what makes you feel good and bad, which foods you like and dislike, and perhaps even whether you like the sea or thunderstorms. The answers to these questions will help reveal your emotional make-up – homeopaths believe that pain is inextricably linked with a person's emotions because neurological pain impulses register in the same part of the brain as emotions.

To find a homeopath who is also a medically qualified doctor, contact the British Homeopathic Association. If you don't mind whether you have a medically qualified homeopath or not, contact the Hahnemann Society or The Society of Homeopaths for details of members in your area who have a particular interest in pregnancy and childbirth. They will have done about three years' full-time training.

If you would like the homeopath to be with you during your labour, phone them and check first whether this is possible. Not all are willing to commit themselves because being with you could mean they have to stay up all night then see their usual quota of patients the next day. Make sure you like and feel comfortable with the practitioner. If you don't, they aren't the right person to be with you during your labour, and it would be best to find another one.

Fees may be a stumbling block. Charges for the initial, in-depth consultation vary, but the average is £35-£60. Subsequent consultations during pregnancy to help prepare your body for labour and recovery afterwards will be shorter and will cost less. Remedies are usually included in the consultation fee. To attend an actual birth, a homeopath may suggest a flat fee of £150-£200, or they may charge by the hour. The latter can mean you end up paying more if your labour lasts many hours.

If your homeopath is unable to be with you in labour,

Your homeopathic birth kit

A typical birth kit might include: Bellis perennis, in case of episiotomy and Caesarean; Arnica to help reduce bleeding; Aconite to help calm fear and panic; Kali phos for exhaustion and feeling you cannot cope; and Caulophyllum for births where the contractions, though strong and painful, are not dilating the cervix.

or you prefer them not to be, ask whether it's possible to contact them for advice if necessary at any time. If something unanticipated comes up during your labour that could be treated homeopathically, it's helpful to know you can get the right advice with just a phone call. You need not feel awkward about phoning during labour – some birth partners are in constant touch with the homeopath throughout the labour, even late at night, and many practitioners fully expect this and are used to it.

If you are making up a birth kit, remedies cost £2-£3 per bottle from suppliers, all of whom will send them by post. Buy remedies in liquid or soft-tablet form. If you're having a home birth – as one in 50 women does each year in Britain – ask your midwife or the head of the midwifery team caring for you what their policy is on homeopathy. You are unlikely to encounter a problem because many midwives are interested in this particular therapy.

Bach Flower Remedies

You have probably seen these little brown bottles in health food shops and chemists, with names such as Rock Rose, Honeysuckle, Larch and Clematis, or you may have used Rescue Remedy before, which is the most famous one. Made from extracts of wild British plants, trees and flowers, distilled in water and preserved with a little brandy, they are similar to homeopathic remedies in that only a tiny trace of their original active ingredient remains. Although they work very gently and subtly, as homeopathic remedies do, they can be surprisingly helpful for both you and your partner in childbirth.

Flower remedies for labour

- Rescue Remedy, for shock, alarm, fear and anxiety. It can be used by both partners for almost all of labour, and also before and after an emergency Caesarean.
- Olive, for exhaustion. It can be helpful if your labour is long and tiring.
- Gentian, which helps people cope with setbacks. These may include changes you have had to make to

how you wanted your labour to be – perhaps you wanted a water birth but ended up needing an epidural.

- Oak, for courage, strength and renewed energy.
- Walnut, for the transition stage.

You can take these remedies every half an hour or so for as long as you need them. Mix four drops in a little water or place two drops directly under your tongue. People have reported feeling better emotionally within just a few minutes.

Hypnotherapy

There is no single, universally agreed definition of hypnotherapy, but it could be described as a type of psychotherapy involving deep relaxation, that helps people use the power of their mind to achieve positive results. According to a major survey carried out by the British Medical Association, it can be effective as a method of pain control in many different situations, from dentistry and surgery to childbirth.

Hypnotherapists believe the mind has several different levels of consciousness or awareness, and that under hypnosis the conscious mind that we use when wide awake is temporarily by-passed, and the subconscious mind becomes more receptive to any positive suggestions we give it.

Hypnosis puts you into a very relaxed state of mind, similar to the way you feel when you're just about to fall asleep. In this state you are able to concentrate intensely, but also to edit out of your conscious mind anything that is distracting or distressing, including pain.

A hypnotherapist can teach you to put yourself into light hypnosis within one or two sessions, after which you strengthen the skill by practising daily so that it can work powerfully for you when you need it in labour. The do-it-yourself approach is how most women use hypnosis for childbirth. Alternatively, you can ask your hypnotherapist to be with you when you're in labour and do the hypnosis for you.

How it works

Although hypnosis is often presented in stage shows as magic, there's nothing magical about it. Natural trance states occur all the time in everyday life. For instance, if you're trying to talk to someone who is immersed in a newspaper or TV programme, they may answer without looking at you, yet later deny ever having spoken at all. This is a good example of the brain's ability to concentrate on something while choosing not to acknowledge or process it consciously, dealing with it on an automatic, or sub-conscious, level instead. The idea behind hypnosis is to programme the mind not to register any information it does not want to know about – and you can do that with pain signals.

'I used it all the way through and it was brilliant. But my concentration slipped when I was pushing Jenny out – it all got too much – and yes, then it did hurt, but only for a very short while. I would definitely use hypnosis again'

Given the fact that hypnosis is often presented to us as entertainment, there are many misconceptions about it. To set the record straight, it will not:

■ Send you to sleep, unless you are trying to actually get to sleep and using hypnotherapy as a way to do so.
■ Make you do anything against your will or better judgement. The hypnotherapist merely gives you suggestions that you may follow or not as you wish. You stay in control of what you do.
■ Make you reveal any secrets. Just as when you are awake, you decide what you are going to reveal and to whom. If hypnotherapy is used as part of psychoanalysis or counselling to help someone speak about a distressing time, it merely makes it easier for the person to talk about it. It will not make them do so against their will.
■ Behave bizarrely or out of character. Self-hypnosis for childbirth cannot make you do or say anything that goes against your common sense or good judgement.

What hypnosis can do is give you control over several

physical functions within your body, from your heart and breathing rate to your perception of pain. For example, under hypnosis you can either relax your muscles or encourage them to work at peak efficiency. Both can be helpful in labour. Relaxation will help counteract the muscular tension in the first and second stages, which tends to create more pain, and encourage peak efficiency in your womb muscles, which will help when you push your baby out. There are many reports from doctors and midwives who have seen it happen, that hypnotherapy can shorten the second stage, too.

'I did a couple of hypnotherapy classes with three other women from my antenatal group. But though I wanted to, I just could not bring myself to believe that something like this could really protect me from pain that bad. And it didn't. I got so worried when the contractions began to hurt so much that I had pethidine as well, and then could not remember my self-hypnosis routine anyway'

Under hypnosis you can also control the amount of pain you feel far better than when in your normal, wide-awake state. It is also possible, using a technique called 'glove hypnosis', to produce a numb feeling in any part of your body so as not to feel any sensation. This has been done so successfully that operations have been performed without any need for general anaesthetic.

Controlling pain using glove hypnosis

In glove hypnosis you are taught how to make one of your hands become totally numb (you may be told to imagine you are plunging your hand into ice-cold water). It is then possible, with practice, to use that hand to pass on the numbness to other parts of the body simply by touching them.

In labour, this technique can be used to numb your abdomen, thereby reducing the pain you feel from contractions. It can also be used when you are pushing your baby out, or to numb the area around your perineum and labia if they need stitches afterwards.

A woman in labour who has mastered the technique

should be able to concentrate deeply on relaxation and ignore some, if not all, of the pain of her contractions.

How you use it

You can be hypnotised by a therapist or they can teach you to hypnotise yourself. It takes a while to learn how to hypnotise yourself, and you need to practise during your pregnancy, as often as you would practise breathing techniques or other relaxation methods. Once you have learned the technique you can use it wherever and whenever you like.

Tell your midwife

Let your midwife and obstetrician know you are using self-hypnosis. Because you will be so calm, you may appear to be in an earlier stage of labour than is the case, and so they will need to check the progress of your labour more carefully. Ideally, you should have vaginal examinations every hour to see how far your cervix has dilated. For comfort, ask to have these carried out while you are lying on your side or standing with one leg raised on a chair, rather than lying on your back. Also, self-hypnosis can, very occasionally, mask problems in labour.

How fast it works

Hypnosis usually takes effect within 20-30 minutes, sometimes sooner, and can last throughout the whole of your labour if you continue to reinforce it.

When you can use it

You can use hypnosis at any stage of your labour. It can also be helpful afterwards for breastfeeding problems, post-delivery pain, the fourth-day blues, and helping you make the most of what sleep you can get with a new baby.

How effective it is

Research has been ongoing internationally since the USA's Stanford University set up its Laboratory of Hypnosis Research in the 1960s. There are now similar projects in

Canada, Australia and Europe. The effect of hypnosis in labour varies. For some women it works so well that they have a virtually pain-free labour. For others it takes the edge off the pain and helps keep them calmer. But for some it is not helpful at all. Generally it is thought that:

- Hypnosis reduces labour pain by about one third.
- Mothers using hypnosis in their labours use less pain-killing medication, sometimes none at all.
- Hypnosis can shorten labour by about one third.

Several small studies support the above. One in 1997 was done at the General Military Hospital in Jinan, China, with 120 first-time mothers. The nurses used psychological suggestion therapy for half of them and found that these mothers had quicker labours. At the USA's University of Wisconsin in 1991, doctors did an experiment involving 60 pregnant women, preparing one group for their childbirths with six hypnosis lessons, and teaching the other group breathing and relaxation techniques. The hypnosis group spent less time in the first stage of labour, used fewer pain-killing drugs and managed to deliver more of their babies without the need for forceps or ventouse than the other group. Their babies were in better shape at birth, too, and had higher Apgar scores (see right).

Another study at the Aberdare District Maternity Unit in Wales in 1993 compared labour in a group of 626 mothers, some of whom had had six hypnotherapy sessions. Of the women who had been hypnotised, those who were giving birth for the first time had much shorter labours than is usual – as short as if for a second or third baby (first labours take about seven to nine hours, subsequent labours on average four to five). The first-time mothers using hypnosis were also three times more likely to be able to cope without any other pain relief than the first-timers who did not use hypnotherapy.

Back in 1986, St George's Hospital, London, carried out a small trial to look at the difference in labour between 29 women who used hypnosis and 36 who did not. Although the women using hypnosis still needed as much drug-based pain relief as the other group, they did have a

The Apgar score

Within a minute of being born, your baby will undergo five checks – pulse/heart rate, breathing, movements, reflexes and skin colour – to assess the physical condition she has arrived in. For each she will be given a score between zero and two. Most babies score between seven and 10.

shorter first stage of labour. And they said that their labour had been a better experience for using hypnosis.

However, in Aberdeen, work with 262 first-time and subsequent mothers in 1994 found that hypnosis *did* reduce the need for pain relief, especially for first-time mothers, and that the first stage of labour was shorter for first-timers. What is more, the hypnosis seemed to have a positive effect on the baby.

Hypnosis has also been used successfully to help prevent premature labour, and even turn around babies who were in the wrong position to be born. In 1986 39 mothers at risk of having their babies too soon were given sessions of hypnotic relaxation, while another group of 70 were given medication. The hypnosis group kept their babies inside them for 'significantly' longer. And in 1994 100 women whose babies were in the breech (bottom-first) position had hypnosis, while another 100 women with breech babies did not. Remarkably, in the hypnosis group, eight out of 10 of the babies either turned themselves the right way around or responded to an obstetrician trying to get them to turn from the outside, but only five out of 10 in the non-hypnosis group managed this.

Hypnotherapy – the pros

- It can reduce labour pain by about one third.
- It may make your labour shorter by about one third.
- It may make a labour *seem* shorter. Under hypnosis, most people's perception of time changes, and usually more time has passed than they realise. And an eight-hour labour that seems like a five-hour one may be no bad thing.
- It's under your own control.
- There are no negative side effects for mother or baby.
- It's drug-free.
- It can be helpful during pregnancy as well as in labour, and its usefulness need not stop after delivery. It can be used for years afterwards to aid sleep and relaxation.
- It's non-invasive.

The power of suggestion
Your subconscious mind will believe almost anything you tell it, including: 'My labour will be comfortable and easy' and 'I am totally relaxed and unworried'.

Hypnotherapy – the cons

- It doesn't work for everyone.
- It takes time to learn and practice.
- You need to find a good hypnotherapist.
- You will have to pay a hypnotherapist to either teach you or be with you in labour.
- Because self-hypnosis can work so successfully, making you feel little pain, your midwife and obstetrician may not think your labour has progressed as far as it has.

How you get it

First, you need to find a professional hypnotherapist with an interest in childbirth to teach you self-hypnosis. Members of The British Society of Medical and Dental Hypnosis are all qualified doctors and dentists. Those of The British Society of Experimental and Clinical Hypnosis are doctors, dentists, graduate psychologists, and sometimes other professionals such as midwives and nurses. And those of The National Register of Hypnotherapists and Psychotherapists are health professionals, such as health workers and psychotherapists (see Resources).

Besides medically qualified hypnotherapists, there are also many lay practitioners (therapists who have no medical background). Their training can be very extensive or it may amount to just a weekend's tuition or even a correspondence course.

More than 80 colleges in the UK offer hypnotherapy diplomas, but it is difficult to know for sure which ones train therapists well and which do not. However, in 1991 Sheffield University became the first in the world to offer a postgraduate diploma course in hypnosis for doctors, dentists and psychologists. London University has now done the same, so a diploma from these colleges is a good sign.

If you would like the therapist to be with you in labour, phone them and check whether this is possible. Then ask about fees. When you meet face to face, see how comfortable you feel – to be able to learn self-hypnosis you must be at ease with your practitioner. If you aren't, find

Positive effect

Always use positive, 'can-do' suggestions when you are programming yourself in hypnosis because the unconscious mind responds better to 'Do's', than to 'Don'ts'. So, 'I will be relaxed and confident' works better than 'I will not be nervous'.

someone else. Once you've found a therapist you like, there are two ways to learn self-hypnosis:

- One-to-one sessions. Just a couple of sessions are enough to learn the methods. A private session with a medically qualified practitioner can cost £35-£80 an hour.
- In groups of between six and 12 women. You would usually need about six sessions. A handful of GPs and hospital antenatal units with an interest in hypnotherapy offer these classes. They may be free or they may have a low flat fee attached.

Course sessions last between one and two hours and, as well as self-hypnosis, you will be taught relaxation methods and probably visualisation techniques to make it more effective.

The self-hypnosis part involves mental exercises designed to put you into a deeply relaxed, receptive state. Once in that state, you then give your mind instructions about how you want your body to behave while under hypnosis – perhaps to feel calm, to feel no pain, or to be unaware of time passing.

When you are practising your hypnosis in the weeks before your labour begins, it can also work very well if you give yourself instructions about how you want your body to behave for the future, after you've come out of hypnosis. This is called post-hypnotic suggestion. One that many pregnant women use is: 'I will have a swift, easy birth'.

The relaxation methods are likely to involve making each part of your body in turn feel heavy, floppy or warm, until you feel loose and relaxed all over. Visualisation is seeing in your mind's eye the things you want to happen in reality, to encourage them to do so. You may be asked to imagine your cervix opening gently, like the petals of a flower unfolding, or your contractions becoming strong and steady, like powerful waves rolling onto the shore. Visualisation can also help you feel calm and secure – perhaps imagine yourself in a place that makes you feel safe and relaxed, such as a much-loved armchair by an open fire.

Get it on tape

It is helpful to have a tape that you can use at home to practise with. Most therapists who give individual tuition will customise one especially for you.

150

If there aren't any courses in your area you could get together a group of women from your antenatal class who are interested in hypnotherapy and arrange group sessions with a therapist, dividing the fee between you. This will keep the cost down, but it's time-consuming.

Massage

Massage is simply beneficial touch (through stroking, pressing, rubbing and kneading) that usually involves working a person's muscles, tendons and ligaments. The word itself comes from either the Greek word *masein*, meaning 'to knead', or the Arabic word *mas'h*, meaning 'to press softly'.

Except where the custom is for the mother to give birth alone, people all around the world massage women in labour. It is probably the oldest therapy known to humankind, and has been used in the Far and Middle East since 3000BC. Massage was very popular in Ancient Greece, and Hippocrates, the Greek physician commonly regarded as the father of medicine, wrote in the 5th Century BC: 'The way to health is to have a scented bath and an oiled massage every day'.

Massage is used to soothe and calm, and to loosen and relax tense muscles. Many complementary therapists, including aromatherapists and osteopaths, use massage in their treatments. And reflexologists and shiatsu practitioners use a form of specific modified touch and pressure in their work, too. Most midwives are happy to rub and massage a woman's back during labour but, because many maternity units are short-staffed, they often don't have the time.

How it works in labour
Massage helps ease labour pain in the following ways:
- By encouraging blood flow to stressed, tired and damaged muscles and combating an increased metabolic rate. As muscles contract, they squeeze the blood vessels that run through them. If the muscles are working hard and contracting over a prolonged period of time, as in

labour, the flow of oxygen-rich blood to them will eventually be restricted. Starved of oxygen (a condition known as ischaemia), the muscles go into painful spasms.

As well as restricting the flow of oxygenated blood, the contracting muscles also restrict the flow of deoxygenated blood out of the area, which takes with it any waste products such as lactic acid that muscles generate when they're working hard. As the waste products build up, it's possible that the muscles' nerve endings may become irritated.

However, this irritation may be caused by another consequence of poor blood flow. If cells within the hard-working muscles become damaged, chemicals called bradykinin and histamine are produced, and it could be these, rather than lactic acid, that affect the nerve endings.

The pain you are feeling is also partly caused by an increase in your metabolic rate. The contraction of your womb muscles speeds up the metabolic rate of all the tissues in the surrounding area, which in turn accelerates the onset of pain.

'It was a loving touch when I needed it'

Massage can help to relieve pain caused by the lack of oxygenated blood and the hyped-up metabolic rate because as your muscles fibres are kneaded, fluid is pushed along them. This encourages the removal of lymph fluid and deoxygenated blood to the kidneys and liver for purification, and the arrival of fresh oxygenated blood to take its place.

■ By reducing muscle tension. A taut muscle begins to relax when you knead it. If a muscle has been stressed and gone into spasm, you can soften it to a certain extent using gentle manipulation and massage.

■ By blocking out pain signals and closing the 'gate' to pain. The idea is based on the Gate theory of pain, which suggests that certain painless sensations can override painful sensations. Impulses from nerves all over your body produced by movement, pain, temperature and touch pass through the dorsal horn area at the base of your spine before being transmitted to your brain. The nerve fibres inside the dorsal horn transmit different types of stimuli at different speeds. A-type nerve fibres carry information faster than C-type fibres. Because touch and pressure sensations travel along A fibres, they reach the brain faster than pain signals, which are carried along by C fibres. And so the former effectively muffle some, if not all, of the latter before they can get to the brain to be registered as pain, thereby partially closing the 'gate' to pain.

If, then, you're getting plenty of sensations from being massaged, this helps to block out the pain you would otherwise be feeling. This works even when the pain impulses are stronger than the pleasurable ones. TENS (p164), water (p169) and water injections (p177) work on the same principle.

■ By helping you to relax. When you are stressed, nervous or anxious, the amount of tension in your muscles increases. This causes a drop in your level of endorphin hormones (your body's natural painkillers), which would normally help to reduce labour pain. The fewer endorphins you have to help you, the more stressed you will become, and the more likely you are to produce a group of chemicals called catecholamines. These are usually produced in the second stage of labour to stimulate the powerful expulsive contractions that push the baby out. If they are made too soon they will disrupt your first-stage contractions, which are designed to shrink the womb and pull up the cervix. This, and the fact that catecholamines are also pain-transmitters in their own right, will increase the amount of pain you feel in labour.

Relaxing will help release more endorphins and stop the production of catecholamines. And massage is an effective, gentle way to help you do that.

■ Changing the amounts of injury chemicals your body releases. Have you ever comforted a child who has banged his knee by rubbing the sore, reddened area? Apart from the comfort touch gives, the actual rubbing

'The one who holds'
Navajo Indians call the woman who helps a mother give birth 'the one who holds'. Her traditional duties include supporting the mother physically – and massaging her.

A fast worker
Massage in the right place can relieve pain within 60 seconds.

encourages the release of endorphins, our natural painkillers, in the affected area and a fall in the level of histamines, the 'damage' chemicals.

Histamines are released as soon as an area is strained or hurt. They have an inflammatory effect that makes the entire area sore and, added to an increased blood flow to the area, makes it turn red. So, by reducing the level of histamines and increasing the level of endorphins in the area, rubbing produces two chemical changes that cause the pain to die away gradually.

How you have it

You can, if you're able, rub the part that hurts yourself but this tends to tense up other parts of your body, and it never feels as good as when someone else does it for you. If no-one is available, it's possible to massage your own back by leaning back against a wall with a tennis ball wedged in between your back and the wall at the point where it hurts. Move up and down and from side to side gently until you get some relief. Wooden-roller massage aids, which you can buy from health shops or chemists, can also be helpful.

But it's best if you can get your partner or midwife to do some massage for you. These general tips will provide some relief:

■ Ask to be rubbed exactly where it hurts. They will need to apply firm pressure and move their hands around a little. If the pressure is in the same place all the time it will make the area sore after a while.

■ Ask to have the top of your shoulders and the back of your neck massaged. Tension often builds up in these areas when you are bracing yourself against the contractions, eventually making them painfully rigid.

■ Have them apply long, firm strokes down each side of your spine using alternate hands. These strokes can extend down your hips and thighs, areas where some women experience considerable pain.

■ Have your buttocks kneaded firmly, as if someone were making dough with them. This provides a helpful counter-pressure to lower-back pain. If your partner's or midwife's hands are getting tired, suggest they use their fists, rolling their knuckles around the buttocks in slow circular movements.

■ Ask for a head and scalp massage. Slow, rhythmical rubbing with firm fingertips in circular strokes all over the scalp and down the back of the neck can feel wonderful. There are many tiny muscles between the skull and the scalp that can become very tense.

Six 'do's' for a labour masseur
■ Use almond oil or plain talcum powder to avoid friction.
■ Always warm the oil in your hands before you use it.
■ Rest your hands gently on the mother's shoulders for 30 seconds before starting.
■ Breathe calmly and deeply as you are massaging – the mother will pick up your relaxed breathing rhythm.
■ While you are pouring more massage oil into your palm, always keep one hand, even if it is just the side or back of it, touching the mother's body so that you do not break contact.
■ As you finish do the last few strokes slower and slower, then rest your hands on the mother's body for 10-20 seconds before taking them away slowly.

Special massage and stretches for labour.
The following techniques are osteopathic and based on gentle supported stretches as well as massage.
■ The lower rib stretch. When you push your baby out you will be using the muscles where the ribs are attached to the thoracic part of her spine. It's important to keep these loose. Sit on a chair or on the edge of your bed with your partner sitting beside you. Have him place one hand on your waist area, on the nearest side to him, and another on your nearest shoulder. Lean gently sideways into him. As you do so, ask him to stretch the area between his hands. Repeat on the other side.

Practise in advance
If your partner would like to massage you during labour, practise techniques and positions beforehand. It is not a good idea to wait until you are in labour – you will be in pain and want immediate relief, and he will be anxious and under pressure to help while having to read notes or a book.

■ The labour rub. This is a very simple and effective massage that can be done as you sit, lie on your side, are on all fours or are leaning across the back of a chair, a pile of cushions or a beanbag, or over the edge of a bath or the rim of a birthing pool. It applies counter-pressure to your sacrum (the base of your back). Your partner needs to massage in rotating circles, crossing his hands over the centre of your lower back and rocking to and fro to use his body weight as he does so.

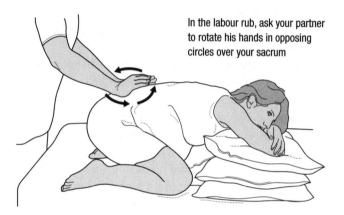

In the labour rub, ask your partner to rotate his hands in opposing circles over your sacrum

■ The whole back stretch. Sit on a chair or on the edge of your bed with your partner standing facing you with one foot in front of the other. Ask him to put his arms around you, passing them underneath your arms, and loosely hold his hands together in the middle of your upper back. Rest your head against his chest, with your hands resting on his upper arms or shoulders. Ask your partner to rock to and fro gently, stretching you upwards for a few seconds each time.

Don't be afraid to tell your partner what feels good and what doesn't, and give instructions such as 'harder' and 'a bit to the left'. This is no time to worry about hurting his feelings, and most people would rather know if they are being helpful or not. Many men are only too willing to massage their partners in labour and are happy to have something specific to do.

How fast it works

Massage can work remarkably quickly, but some types work faster than others. A general neck and shoulder massage for relaxation should start to relax you and reduce pain within about 10 minutes. But if someone is rubbing firmly on a particular area that is hurting, this could begin to help within a minute or two. The relaxation it brings can last for some time after the massage is over, too.

When you can, and can't, have it

You can have massage at any stage of labour. If, however, you are having a Caesarean with a standard epidural, your partner will be able to massage only your head, hands and the front of your shoulders, as you will be reclining.

Many women find touch comforting and helpful in their labours. Others find it irritating and just want to be left alone, particularly in the transition stage. You can't predict how you'll feel, and your feelings might even change at different points in your labour.

How effective it is

About 10% of women use massage in labour, with massage defined as specific and special techniques rather than general rubbing for a brief period. Although most midwives will rub a woman's lower back at intervals if they have time, this comes under the heading of 'brief, general rubbing' and is often more of a kindly, supportive gesture of encouragement than a concerted effort to reduce pain.

In the National Birthday Trust Survey of 1990, which looked at all the methods then available of relieving pain in childbirth in the UK, nine out of 10 mothers said they found a 'proper' massage was a 'good' or 'very good' method of pain relief.

Lower-back massage and pressure seems to be especially helpful for women who are feeling most of the pain in their lower back. These types of labours are called 'back labours' and can cause considerable pain that can be quite difficult to soothe.

A study in 1981 at the Obstetrics and Gynaecology

Massage with an epidural
If you have had a standard epidural, stiffness and tension can still build up in your upper body. Because it's more difficult to have your lower back massaged, ask your partner to do your hands and head instead. If you have feeling in your feet, ask him to rub these, too. These areas have plenty of nerve endings and many reflexology (p159) and acupressure points (see Acupuncture, p102).

Unit of Grand Rapids Osteopathic Hospital in Michigan, USA, looked at 500 women in labour who had particular back pain, and found that in 87% of cases it was associated with their babies lying in awkward positions. The staff tried osteopathic techniques and lower-back massage for half of them. For the other half, staff massaged less appropriate areas of the back. Of the group receiving true lower-back massage, 81% said it helped. And, in fact, the group that received massage to the 'wrong' areas of the back needed about 30% more pain-killing drugs and 50% more of the tranquillising drugs that are often used for labour in the USA.

'To my surprise, I found it got on my nerves – so I slapped his hands away (I was beyond speech by that time)'

Massage – the pros
- It can be very effective.
- It can start working within 60 seconds.
- It is comforting in other ways, not just as a method of pain relief. Sympathetic touch encourages closeness, a feeling of physiological and psychological support, and improved communication between the mother and those around her.
- It is easily available and free.
- It is non-invasive.
- It is drug-free.
- There are no side effects for mother or baby.

Massage – the cons
- You need to have someone else do it for you.
- The person who massages you may not do it very well or for as long as you would like them to.
- You can practise massage for labour for weeks beforehand with your partner and then, when it comes to the time, you may not want to be touched.

How you get it
The massage will work best if you practise with your

partner or birth companion before your baby is due. Experiment with the techniques and suggestions in this section. Classes run by The National Childbirth Trust and the Active Birth Centre will also cover massage (see Resources).

Reflexology

Sometimes known as zone therapy, reflexology involves gently manipulating and pressing certain areas of the feet and hands to help correct illness, soothe pain and calm the mind. In the same way that acupuncturists may treat women in labour by inserting needles only into the ear, reflexology is based on a similar principle – that a small area of the body can be a microcosm of the whole. As such, it can be used to bring about changes, sometimes powerful, in parts of the body that have not been touched directly.

Reflexologists believe that the hands and feet are energy maps of the rest of you, and that there are areas on the hands, face and feet called reflex points which are directly linked to each organ and structure within the body. They also believe that the body is divided into 10 vertical zones, five on the left and five on the right. Each zone runs from your head down to the reflex points in your hands and feet, and from the front through to the back of your body. All body parts within each zone are thought to be linked by nerve pathways to the soles of your feet or your hands. So, your left and right pelvic areas and your sciatic nerve are linked to your heels, and your sexual and reproductive organs are linked to your ankles.

No-one is entirely sure how reflexology works beyond the act of stimulating the nerve endings in the hands and feet (there are 14,000 in the soles of your feet alone). One explanation is that there is a fine network of weak electrical energy (like *qi* in traditional Chinese medicine and acupuncture) that flows continuously along the body's nerve pathways. Certainly, the presence of electrical energy has been confirmed by Western electrical engineering scientists investigating acupuncture (see References).

Work on your ankle
Reflexologists believe there is a point on the inside of your ankle that connects directly to your womb. By pressing and rubbing it gently it's possible to soothe period pain and certain types of labour pain.

Reflexologists say that your wellbeing depends on that energy being free to move around uninterrupted, and that if any of its routes become blocked, pain or health problems will affect the area it would normally be supplying.

Another theory is that reflexology works because of the mechanical pressure of the fingers pressing or rubbing on specific areas, sending out small pulses of bio-electrical energy that helps clear blockages and restore a normal, uninterrupted energy flow.

It is thought that pain in labour can be reduced if a therapist works gently over the whole of both feet, but pays special attention to the areas that link to the womb, pituitary gland, lymphatic system and pelvic organs.

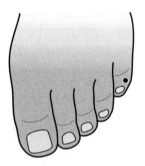

To relieve labour pain and encourage your contractions to be efficient, try pressing the Zhiyan point on the outside of your little toe (shown left)

How it works in labour

As well as stimulating energy flow to the areas of your body that are hurting, there is evidence to suggest that reflexology stimulates the body's production of hormones. These may include the ones that drive your labour (oxytocin) and your natural painkillers (endorphins). Some British midwives and nurses use reflexology in their practices. From their comments and those of mothers, it appears that reflexology can indeed be helpful for pain relief, cervical dilation and speeding up labour – all processes that are controlled by hormones.

The gentle massage involved in a treatment offers other benefits in labour, too, helping you to relax and focus your mind.

How fast it works

If you have professional reflexology during your labour it can start working within a minute or two. Its full benefits are felt after about 15 minutes and can last for an hour or two (you can have more reflexology if and when you need it). You may still be getting some lesser beneficial effects as much as 24-48 hours later.

When you can use it

You can use reflexology in any stage of labour. If you are having a Caesarean, your therapist – or your partner if he has been shown how – can work on the points on your hands rather than those on your feet.

How effective it is

Like most methods of pain relief, especially complementary methods, the effects of reflexology vary. However, it has been reported that many women using reflexology have needed no additional pain relief, and that midwives who have used this technique say first-time mothers had 'better than expected' labours as a result.

Several studies on reflexology in labour, the results of which have been published in East European and Russian medical journals, suggest it can be helpful for soothing pain in the first stage (see References). And an article entitled 'Reflex Zone Therapy for Mothers' published in *Nursing Times* in 1990 also concluded that reflexology was helpful for women in labour.

Promising work using reflexology in general pain management was carried out in the 1990s by Cambridge University with staff from Ely Hospital. And one particular British study of 64 first-time mothers in 1992-3 found that reflexology in pregnancy reduced the need for additional pain relief in labour and produced quicker, problem-free births. It also seemed to help a wide range of pregnancy problems, such as heartburn and raised blood pressure.

That study was carried out by Dr Gowrie Mowtha, a private London GP and reflexologist with a special interest

Reflexology and Caesareans
In 1984 a team of Russian obstetricians carried out a series of Caesarean deliveries using only reflexology and a light anaesthetic.

161

in natural childbirth and natural pain relief. Of the mothers who had 10 reflexology sessions beginning in the middle of their pregnancies, only 2.7% had an epidural (the national average is about 20%). The first stage of labour took about five hours, shorter than the national average. And the second stage of labour, which usually takes between one and two hours, took an average of about 16 minutes.

'I'd had reflexology before for a minor complaint so was confident that it could help with labour, too – I only used it at the beginning, but I'm sure it helped make the first stage quicker'

Interestingly, the little UK clinical research that has been, or is being, done on reflexology also looks at the effect it has on reproductive hormones, except that these studies concentrate on areas such as premenstrual syndrome (PMS) and infertility problems. The in vitro fertilisation (IVF) unit at Derriford Hospital in Plymouth is currently running a trial using reflexology to improve and stabilise the level of ovulation hormones in patients, with the effect of the treatments being checked and measured by regular blood tests. And a study in 1991 at the University of California in Los Angeles showed weekly reflexology treatments reduced PMS symptoms by 62%. Again, the doctors running the research thought the reflexology had possibly helped by modifying hormone levels.

DIY reflexology
Ask your therapist to show your partner some basic points he can work on for you in labour. If he doesn't get the opportunity to be shown these, he can still help by giving you a simple foot massage to help warm your feet. Women in labour often have cold feet because their energy is being directed elsewhere.

Reflexology – the pros
- It can work fast.
- It may be very effective.
- You can do it yourself – or your partner can be shown how.
- It is relaxing and calming in its own right.
- You do not need to buy any special equipment or substances (for instance, with aromatherapy you need to buy essential oils, and with TENS you need the small electrical unit).
- It's non-invasive, unlike acupuncture, which works on similar principles but which involves the use of needles.

- It is drug-free.
- It may be useful for other labour problems, such as helping your womb work more efficiently, which reduces labour pain in itself. Newborn babies apparently like it, too (ask your reflexologist for one or two points to press gently for your baby).

Reflexology – the cons
- It may not work for you.
- It's very important that a properly qualified therapist treats you or shows you or your partner some points to work on.
- You have to pay for advice from a qualified therapist.
- It can be expensive to have a reflexologist with you throughout your childbirth.
- Your hospital may not be keen for you to have a therapist with you in labour.

How you get it
To find a professionally qualified reflexologist, contact the Institute of Complementary Medicine or the Association of Reflexologists (see Resources). If you would like a reflexologist to be with you during your labour, negotiate a flat fee rather than an hourly rate, which could work out as very expensive. Expect to pay £150-£250. Not all therapists are willing to be with a woman in labour as they may have to stay up through the night and/or cancel other clients at the last minute. If you'd just like one or two sessions, with guidance on reflexology for labour, expect to pay £25-£45 for the first session. This should include an interview in which your medical history is taken, a treatment, and instruction on which reflex points should be pressed for pain relief in labour.

If you are having your baby in hospital, check with the Head of Midwifery Services that there will be no problem about having your therapist with you in a professional capacity. It is safest to do this several weeks in advance of your due date in case the hospital refuses and you have to argue your case or find another hospital.

Easy reflexology rub
Ask your partner or midwife to hold each of your heels in turn between both of their hands and rub vigorously. Because your heels are linked to the whole of your pelvic area, this can help ease labour pains and encourage your womb to work more efficiently.

Transcutaneous Electrical Nerve Stimulation (TENS)

TENS is a method of pain relief that involves the use of four small electrode pads that deliver a very mild electrical stimulus to your lower back. This stimulus can help reduce the pain of contractions during labour by stopping some of the pain signals from your womb reaching your brain.

The TENS machine is small and light – about the size of a cigarette packet – with a push-button boost control. Because it is battery-operated it's easy to walk around and change positions with it on. TENS is also helpful for backache before and after you give birth. Several other versions of the system are used in the NHS to relieve post-operative discomfort and to help deal with certain types of chronic pain, including arthritis, neuralgia, sciatica and pain from damage to the back's discs.

'It was good for the early to middle stages, but it did not seem to really touch the later stage at all. Also, the electrode pads and wires got in the way of my husband massaging my back'

TENS is thought to work in two ways:

■ Electrical stimulation at a rate of 2 Hertz (pulses) a second is thought to stimulate the release of endorphins (your body's own pain-killing hormones), traces of which have been found in the fluid that bathes the spinal cord. TENS is said to raise the body's endorphin levels if you start using it early on in labour, while the pain is mild.

■ During first-stage contractions the electrical impulses from the TENS machine travel along fast-conducting A fibres to the brain, arriving there ahead of the pain impulses from your contracting womb, which travel along the slow-conducting C fibres. This is called the Gate theory of pain (see p152 for a full explanation). The TENS stimuli are closing the 'gate' to pain by overriding the pain impulses reaching the brain.

How you use it

To use a TENS machine first place one pair of electrodes (they are on self-adhesive pads) about halfway up your back on either side of your spine, and the other pair parallel to them on either side of the base of your spine, just above your buttocks. It is possible to put them on yourself, but easier if a friend, your partner or your midwife does it for you. If you are not quite sure where to place the electrodes, take them to your final antenatal appointment and ask a midwife to mark four 'X's on your back with an indelible pen showing where they need to go. You can practise putting them on looking over your shoulder in a full-length mirror.

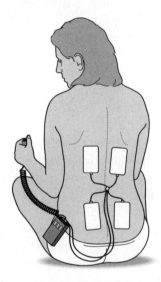

With TENS, four electrode pads are stuck on your back. You control how much stimulus you feel using the dials on the machine and the boost button you hold in your hand

It is a good idea to try out the TENS machine before you need it, so you can get used to using it and also to the sensation it produces. Try wearing it for half a day, and practise with the settings and pressing the boost button each time you have a Braxton Hicks contraction. Many women also use it to help soothe nagging backache late in their pregnancy, which for some can become severe and make it difficult to sleep.

Start using TENS as soon as your contractions become uncomfortable so its effects can build up as much as possible to help you as your labour progresses. Apart from

Natural painkillers
Endorphins, the natural painkillers that your own body produces, are many times stronger than morphine.

165

encouraging your own natural pain-killing hormones to build up in your system, there is another reason for starting TENS as early as possible. If you wait too long, repeated pain stimuli travelling along your neurological pathways will have increased the pathways' responsiveness to pain, making you more sensitive to it, possibly so much so that when TENS is eventually used you will not find it much help.

'I didn't think it was doing much. So I stopped pressing the boost button for the next couple of contractions, and immediately realised just how much it had been helping after all'

Preventing this potentially heightened sensitivity is called pain prophylaxis. It is recommended by many top anaesthetists and pain experts, including a consultant anaesthetist at University College Hospital who, following the same principle, recommends that people take a painkiller *before* they have a filling at the dentist's rather than after.

You can adjust the TENS machine to deliver high, medium and low doses of stimulation, depending on how much pain relief you need. At its lowest setting you may feel a constant gentle buzzing or mild tingling. If you increase the level of stimulation this will increase, along with any pain-relieving effects. As you turn it up further the buzzing becomes stronger and, unless you are having a contraction, it can start to feel a bit uncomfortable.

An ancient remedy
Electricity has been used in medicine since AD46 when the Roman doctor Scribonius Largos used an electric ray (a member of the stingray family) to treat headache and gout. The shock from the ray stimulated the affected area and apparently helped to relieve some of the pain.

Leave the machine on all the time while you are in labour, turning it up gradually as your contractions become stronger. Press the boost button each time a contraction begins, to give yourself a bit more stimulation, then press it again to stop the extra stimulation as each one finishes.

The machine's makers recommended that you continue using it for an hour or two after your baby has been born to help keep your endorphin levels up. This may help soothe any discomfort you have, perhaps because you have had stitches (some women say being stitched hurts more than the birth itself) or because of general tissue stretching and soreness.

166

How fast it works

TENS begins to take effect almost immediately if you start using it early. You will feel its full effects within about half an hour, as it takes endorphin levels this long to build up. Once established, they take some time to clear from your system, so the pain-relieving effects of TENS can last for a while after the electrical stimulation stops. If the machine has been on long enough to generate a high enough level of endorphins, the pain-killing effect will continue for an hour or so after it is switched off.

When you can, and can't, use it

It's best to use TENS in the early part of labour. About 75% of women who initially found it helpful say it didn't give effective relief in the second stage. This is thought to be because, unlike in the first stage of labour, when pain signals can be overridden by the electrical impulses of the TENS machine, the pain signals in the second stage of labour cannot. This is because they come more from the birth canal and the perineum, and travel mostly along the fast-conducting A fibres, down which the TENS impulses also travel, reaching the brain at the same time. One cannot, therefore, override the other one.

'Very good. I was able to cope until the late stages without gas, and so felt I was more in control'

You cannot use TENS if you have a heart pacemaker, if your baby's heart rate is being monitored electronically, or if you are in water. Nor can the electrodes be put on areas of skin that are broken or irritated. Check with an acupuncturist whether you can use TENS if you are having electro-acupuncture.

How effective it is

Estimates vary widely as to the effectiveness of TENS. Some trials suggest it's 70-80% effective, others suggest it's no help at all. Obstetricians are usually pretty scathing about it. Many regard it as 'essentially a labour-saving but fairly expensive way of rubbing someone's back'. It is

Other options

TENS can be good for calming pain in the first stage of labour, but it's usually no help in the second stage, when you are pushing your baby out. Many women use gas and air instead then or, if available, a nerve block. This is a pain-killing injection that provides relief exactly where you need it (see Paracervical block, p88, and Pudendal block, p92).

not very popular in the USA, yet mothers in the UK and other European countries like it better. Interestingly, women themselves and their midwives seem to rate TENS higher than doctors do.

TENS – the pros

- It is drug-free and non-invasive.
- It can be used from the very beginning of labour. This may mean you are able to stay at home for longer before going to hospital.
- It is good for using at home births.
- It can be very effective.
- It is helpful for backache before and after labour, too.
- Once correctly attached to your back, it is in your control.
- You can increase its effect immediately if you need to.
- There are no reported side effects for mother or baby.
- It does not affect your awareness.
- You can move about as much as you like.
- It is compatible with other forms of pain relief, except water and possibly electro-acupuncture (check with your acupuncturist).
- It can be useful when you have an internal examination to check how far your cervix has opened.
- If you do not like it, you can take it off immediately.

TENS – the cons

- You may find it's no help at all.
- It does not usually work in the second stage of labour.
- Wires can get in the way of back massage.
- If used for a long period, TENS can cause some skin irritation around the site of the electrodes.
- You may have to switch the machine off if any electronic fetal monitoring is taking place.
- Some women dislike the sensation it produces, although many who initially find it irritating say they no longer notice it once they start having painful contractions.

How to get it

About 50% of maternity units have TENS machines, but

many have only one or two, which means they may be in use when you need one. Ask what the situation is at your hospital. If you are having a home birth, ask if your midwife has one. Alternatively, hire a machine for a month for about £25 (see Resources for stockists) or buy one.

If money is a problem, you could share one with another mother, perhaps someone you know from your antenatal classes, whose baby is not due in the same week as yours.

Spare battery
Always keep a spare battery handy in case the one in your TENS machine runs out while you are using it in labour.

Water

Everyone knows about the relaxing and pain-relieving effects of a warm bath, so it's no surprise that many women in labour are instinctively drawn to water. While an ordinary bath or shower can be helpful, for water to have the maximum effect it's best to use a purpose-built birthing pool. These should be deep enough for the water to come up to breast level when you are kneeling in it, and big enough for a second person to get in there with you if necessary. Many companies offer specially designed pools for hire, and eight out of 10 UK hospitals now have their own.

Merely changing your environment – in this case, from dry land to water – is often enough to affect the way your labour is progressing. This effect can sometimes be seen in women who arrive at hospital in full labour only to find their labour suddenly slows to a halt. However, when water is used, the effect on labour is often for the better – many women whose labours are not progressing well notice improvements as soon as they get into a warm pool or bath. Similarly, if labour is going very slowly or has stopped progressing for a woman who is in water, getting out can reverse the situation.

Using water to ease labour pain and actually giving birth in water are two different things. Many water enthusiasts believe giving birth in water is a gentle, safe and natural way to introduce a baby into the world. While water births are perfectly safe (research over the past 10 years shows it's just as safe to give birth in a pool as it is on dry land if you are a 'low-risk' mother, as most are), many of the women who use pools still prefer to get out to deliver their baby. Women who have given birth in water talk about the pleasure, satisfaction and security that water births offer, and some even remember it as being a powerfully sensual experience. For more detailed information on giving birth in water, contact the Active Birth Centre (see Resources).

'It was just the best night of my life'
North London NHS paediatrician
Caroline Fertleman talking about the labour
and birth of her third child in a birthing pool

How it works in labour
There are many reasons why being in warm water soothes labour pain:
■ Relaxation. The feel and warmth of the water, and the support it gives you, will help you relax physically and mentally, reducing the pain you feel.
■ As the water makes you more relaxed, your system will produce more endorphins (powerful natural painkillers and mood uplifters), and may also help stimulate strong womb contractions.
■ You are more mobile in water and can change position easily. This can help you feel more comfortable.
■ You feel lighter, which is a pleasant contrast to how you have been feeling on dry land recently, with the full force of gravity pulling you down.
■ The feel of water all over your body can help block out pain signals. The idea is based on the Gate theory of pain, which suggests that it's possible for some painless sensations to override painful sensations (see p152 for a full explanation of Gate theory).
■ There is less pressure on your abdomen, which will encourage your womb to contract more efficiently and improve your blood circulation, resulting in more oxygen getting to your womb muscles. If the muscles are starved of oxygen they go into spasm, which hurts. If they have a good supply of oxygen, they will hurt less.

■ Privacy, peace and quiet. This can be very important to women in labour, but it may be in short supply in a busy NHS unit. If you are in hospital, the birthing pool will be in its own quiet room. And even if you can only have a bath or shower, you will be away from the main bustle of the labour ward. If you have a bit of privacy you are more likely to relax because you feel protected, and also because you have some space which is yours alone, and this in itself can reduce the pain you feel.

■ You may be less likely to need an episiotomy. This may be partly because your tissues stretch more easily in warm water, and partly because it is more difficult for your midwife or obstetrician to do one if you are in water. There is plenty of research that supports this. One of the most recent studies, in Switzerland, looked at 2000 water births and found that only one in 10 mothers who had their baby in water needed an episiotomy, compared to one in three mothers who had their baby on a special birth bed.

How you have it

Your obstetrician or midwife may advise you to wait until you are 5cm dilated before getting into the pool. This is because if you get in sooner, before labour is in full swing, you may become a bit too relaxed and your oxytocin output can drop, which will either slow your contractions right down or even stop them altogether. This isn't usually that much of a problem though, as things should get going again once you get out of the water, but it can mean that your labour progresses in a bit of a stop/start way instead of smoothly and continuously.

Medical staff usually regard labour as being well established – that is, well under way and fairly unstoppable – when you are having regular strong contractions about 10 minutes apart and your cervix has dilated to 5cm. However, it can be hard to wait, and many women would prefer to get into the pool sooner.

While waiting to get into the birthing pool, try using other pain-relieving techniques, such as distraction

In this together
Three out of four husbands and boyfriends get into the pool with their partner once labour is under way.

therapy, breathing, autogenic training, self-hypnosis, TENS, relaxation and visualisation, reflexology, aromatherapy and massage. If you find you are really craving some contact with water, try a warm shower, which can be surprisingly calming and soothing in its own right. Change position as often as you like, move about as much as you want, and stay upright or semi-upright as much as you can.

When you do get into the pool, it's important to have the water at the right depth. It should cover your belly, yet leave your shoulders exposed so you can lose heat if you need to. Your partner can top it up if necessary.

Once you are in the water you can still use some other methods of pain relief, including homeopathy, massage, self-hypnosis, yoga, breathing and relaxation, reflexology and ear acupuncture (but not electro-acupuncture). You will not be able to use TENS in the water either, but you can if you get out and are dried properly.

Some midwives and doctors are happy for you to use gas and air, too, if you want it. But it may make you dizzy and at risk of slipping if you move around in the pool while you are taking it. If you want to use it, discuss it with your midwife and perhaps try it to see how you get on.

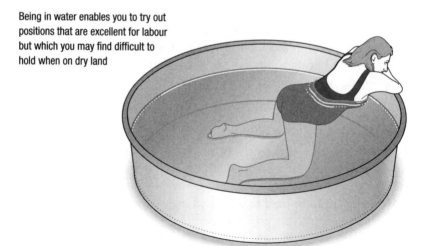

Being in water enables you to try out positions that are excellent for labour but which you may find difficult to hold when on dry land

You will need a canister of the gas mounted on wheels, and you should not be left alone in case you do suddenly feel dizzy or faint.

How fast it works

The water will start to take effect in about the same time it takes for a warm bath to relax you after a hard day. You will feel the full effects in 10-20 minutes, and they'll last for as long as you remain in the water. Some of the calming effect may even continue after you leave the water.

When you can, and can't, have it

Because most hospitals have birthing pools, and it's relatively easy to hire one for home use, labouring in water is an option that's open to most women. There are certain circumstances where it won't be possible to use water:
■ The hospital pool may already be in use when you need it.
■ If you are in very early labour. Your midwife or doctor will probably advise you to wait for a while.
■ If your baby needs continuous heart monitoring. This is necessary when there are signs that the baby is in distress, such as an abnormally rapid fetal heartbeat or meconium (the greenish waste that's your baby's first bowel movement) in your waters when they break. Only one method of continuous monitoring, called telemetry, can be used under water but it is not widely available.
■ If you are suffering from severe pre-eclampsia with very high blood pressure.
■ If you have had any drug-based pain relief, such as pethidine. Because it can make you unsteady on your legs, there's a risk you may slip. However, your midwife and obstetrician may allow you to use gas and air.

How effective it is

Being in water does not offer complete pain relief in the conventional sense, in the way a spinal does. What it does

No problem
Most women move their bowels a little during labour. If this happens while you are in your pool, it can be removed straightaway with an ordinary domestic sieve kept next to the pool for this purpose.

When to get in and out

The golden rule for labour in water is that if things are going slowly when you are *out* of the pool, get into it. If progress is slow *in* the water, get out.

is calm you, encourage you to relax deeply, and reduce the pain you feel to manageable levels. You may even find you do not need any other form of pain relief.

According to Janet Balaskas, a pioneer of water birth and natural childbirth: 'The buoyancy of the water helps support you, and the sensuality of being in warm water helps you to tune into the instinctive consciousness that allows birth to happen.

'What happens is that the pain remains challenging but it is easier to cope with it. You can experience the sensations at the peak of a contraction as intensity of feeling rather than pain, and are able to open up and go with it rather than resist it.'

Water – the pros

- It's usually very calming as well as pain-relieving.
- It can help speed up your labour if it isn't progressing very well.
- It gives you privacy. You cannot put a birthing pool, or even a bath, anywhere except in its own room.
- You may be less likely to need an episiotomy.
- It can reduce heightened blood pressure because it makes you calmer and more relaxed.
- The moist atmosphere in a room with a pool in it makes it easier to breathe (most maternity units are often very dry and overheated). This can be especially helpful for women with asthma.
- Many women say they do not notice time passing when they are in water, and that 'the world beyond the rim of the pool seems to disappear'. This helps you concentrate on working through your contractions without distraction and can make you feel safe. One woman described it as, 'being in my own womb of water'.
- It helps you feel comfortable in upright positions that encourage easier labour, and the water's buoyancy helps you stay in these for longer. Even women who find it difficult to squat (an excellent position as it opens up the pelvis and makes more space for the

baby's head) usually find they can do so in water.

- Checks on your temperature and pulse can still be done without difficulty. A thermometer can be used in the usual way, and your blood pressure can be checked if you stand up (your blood pressure when you stand will be different from your blood pressure if you are sitting, lying or floating, and your midwife will need to take this into account).

Water – the cons

- It doesn't offer total pain relief.
- If your pool doesn't have its own heater and thermostat someone will have to be available to monitor the water temperature and top up the pool with warm water when necessary.
- It's not always possible to monitor your baby continuously. If your hospital does not have a special underwater monitor you will have to get out of the pool. Intermittent monitoring is not a problem as Sonicaid make a monitor suitable for occasional checks under water. Or you can get out of the pool temporarily, or even stand or squat, leaning slightly forward over the pool's rim supported by your arms so that your abdomen is above the waterline (this may be uncomfortable if the monitoring goes on for long).
- You have to pay if you have to hire your own pool.
- A midwife who is not familiar with labour in water may be concerned about her back when having to bend over to look after you, and so may not be keen for you to use a pool. However, there are recommended positions and techniques for those helping women in birthing pools (see Resources).
- Examinations to check how your labour is progressing can be awkward. Your midwife will need to bend over the pool and put her hand and arm under the water as far as her shoulder to feel how far your cervix has dilated. However, if you can float on your back against the side of the pool this shouldn't be too much of a problem.

Safety first

If you are using a birthing pool you must always have someone with you, regardless of whether you have had any pain-relieving drugs.

How you get it

About 150 hospitals in the UK offer a birthing pool, and of the ones that don't, most will be happy for you to hire one and bring it in with you. Check beforehand whether this is permitted and ask whether the unit's floor is structurally strong enough to support it.

Pools are available from several companies for £150-£250 for four weeks (see Resources). You can hire one for a home birth, too. They come in different sizes and have different features. Some have their own heater and thermostat to keep the temperature of the water at a constant level, while others have to have hot water added, which means your pool may take several hours to get ready before you are able to use it. Someone will also have to be on hand to top it up with warm water throughout your labour. It pays to think carefully about what you'd like beforehand.

'Having spent a fair bit of money on a hired pool then, with some difficulty, persuaded the hospital to let me bring it in, I found I was perfectly comfortable with one of the beanbags they had there and I didn't want to move from it. I never even got into the water'

If a pool isn't available to you, staff may suggest you have a bath or shower instead. These options are better than nothing and it may help to try them, but while baths will provide warm water, they lack both the room to manoeuvre and the depth for buoyancy. And while a shower offers warm water, too, it can only be applied to a small area of your body at a time, and it doesn't offer the buoyancy and relaxation of a pool.

If your hospital doesn't have a pool and won't allow you to bring in your own, write to the hospital's Director of Midwifery Services. If they are not receptive, write to the Unit General Manager. If you still have no luck, you may have to find another hospital. Ask local midwives if they can suggest anywhere, or contact the Active Birth Centre, which has a list of hospitals that have a pool. Or contact one of the campaigning childbirth organisations, such as the Association for Improvements in the Maternity

Services or The National Childbirth Trust, who can advise you (see Resources).

Water injections

Also known as lumbar reflexology, water injections are used specifically for back pain in labour. They involve having two small injections of plain sterile water in your lower back, on either side of the base of the spine.

Water injections are thought to work in a similar way to TENS (p164). They form a small temporary area of water that puts pressure on the back's dorsal nerves, which run along the spine, interrupting pain signals travelling from your lower back to your brain. At best they block out all the back pain, at worst none at all.

Getting the injections in the right spot is the key to success, according to water birth initiator Dr Michel Odent. He was also the first doctor to use this method of soothing back pain in labour nearly 30 years ago at his revolutionary maternity hospital in Pithiviers, France. The correct place on the back is just below the last rib, in the little muscular depression on either side of the base of the spine. The injections need to be done into the skin (intracutaneously) and not, as is sometimes done, underneath its fatty layer (subcutaneously).

'I liked the idea of these, but my midwife had never even heard of them'

How fast they work

When the injections are correctly given, they start working within seconds, and take full effect within 30-45 minutes. Since the water is gradually absorbed into the body, the injections may need to be repeated after a few hours, depending on how you are feeling.

How effective they are

The effect of water injections can depend on how accurately they are done. When the areas of water interrupt all the pain signals getting to the brain, you'll be pretty comfortable. If only some of the signals are interrupted, you'll feel less pain but still be conscious of some discomfort. And if the injections aren't in the right place, they won't interrupt any pain signals and will be of no help at all.

Water injections may sound like a fake treatment but they do seem to work and have long been used to beat severe back ache caused by acute kidney pain and a form of appendicitis. In a trial involving 99 women with back pain in labour, carried out by Sweden's University of Skovode, water injections helped ease the back labour pain considerably and were four to five times more effective than dummy injections given in the wrong place.

When you can, and can't, have them

Water injections can be given at any point during labour, but you are highly unlikely to be offered them in the UK. Midwives and obstetricians have not been trained to give the injections, and most are not convinced that they work anyway.

This may be because, as Dr Odent suggests, 'the method is just too simple – it's just water after all', and there are no profits to be made by drug companies, which are usually responsible for funding the clinical trials for new treatments. Water injections are, however, used in Canada, Germany, Sweden, Finland and Denmark, especially by midwives for women who want to have as natural a birth as possible.

Water injections – the pros

- They can be highly effective at relieving back pain in labour.
- They start working immediately, and take full effect within 30-45 minutes.
- The effect lasts up to several hours.
- They are drug-free.
- They are easy to give.

Water injections – the cons
- They are not effective at relieving abdominal pain in labour.
- They are not readily available in the UK.
- You will feel a very brief but stinging pain as the injections are given.

References

Preventing perineal tears
Massage doesn't make much difference – Stamp G, Kruzins G: 'Perineal massage in labour and prevention of perineal trauma: a randomised controlled trial', *BMJ*, May 2001 (Note: the massage was only done in labour, not for a few weeks beforehand as is recommended).
Home birth reduces the rate/hands and knees birth position – Murphy P, Baker Feinland J: 'Perineal Outcomes in a Home Birth Setting', *Birth*, 25/4/1998.

Mothers and babies remembering labour and birth
Niven CA, Murphy-Black T: 'Memory for Labour Pain: a Review of the Literature', *Birth*, 27/4/2000. Rofe Y, Algom A: 'Accuracy of remembering post delivery pain', *Percept Mot Skills*, 1985 (60). Niven C, Brodie E: 'Memory for Labour Pain', *Pain*, 1995 (64). Oates R, Forrest D: 'Reliability of Mothers' Reports of Birth Data', *Austral Paediatr J*, 1984 (20).

Babies' awareness of their mothers' labour and their own birth
Bradford N: *The Miraculous World of Your Unborn Baby*, 2nd ed, Chrysalis Books, 2001. Dr Chamberlain DB: 'The Significance of Birth Memories', *Int J Pre and Perinatal Med*, Summer 1988. Dr Chamberlain DB: 'Reliability of Birth Memory: Observations from Mother & Child in

Pains in Hypnosis', *J Amer Acad Medical Hypnoanalysts*, Dec 1986. Cheek DB: 'Prenatal and Perinatal Imprints: Apparent Prenatal Consciousness as Revealed by Hypnosis', *Int J Pre and Perinatal Psych & Med*, 1986 (vol 1/2). Emerson W: *Infant and Childbirth Refacilitation*, Human Potential Resources, Petaluma, USA, 1984. Laibow RE: 'Birth Recall, a Clinical Report', *Int J Pre and Perinatal Psych & Med*, 1986 (vol 1, no 1). Verny T: *The Secret Life of Your Unborn Child*, Warner Books, 1993.

Unborn babies' awareness of their mothers' emotions
Dr Cheek DB: 'Are Telepathy, Clairvoyance and Hearing Possible In Utero? Suggested evidence as revealed during hypnotic age-regression studies of prenatal memory,' *Int J Pre and Perinatal Psych & Med*, Winter 1992. Correia IB: *The Impact of Television Stimuli on the Prenatal Infant*, doctorate dissertation, Univ of New South Wales, Australia. Prof Hepper P: *The Links Between Maternal Anxiety and Foetal Behaviour*, report at the biennial meeting of the Marce Society, London, Sept 1996. Rossi N: 'Maternal Stress and Fetal Motor Behaviour', *Int J Pre and Perinatal Psych & Med*, 1989 (vol 3, no 4). Van den Bergh BRH: 'The Influence of Maternal Emotions During Pregnancy on Fetal and Neonatal Behaviour', *Int J Pre and Perinatal Psych & Med*, Winter 1990.

Epidurals
Patchy effect – Peach MJ, Godkin R et al: 'Complications of obstetric epidural analgesia and anaesthesia – a prospective analysis of 10,995 cases', *Int J Obst Anaesth*, 1998 (7).
Shivering – Webb PJ et al: 'Shivering during epidural analgesia in women in labor', *Anaesthesiology*, 1981 (55).
Dural puncture at night – Aya AGM et al: 'Increased risk of unintentional dural puncture in night-time obstetrics for epidural anesthesia', *Can J Anaesth*, 1999 (46).
Figs on incidence of dural puncture headache – O'Sullivan G, conslt anaesth, St Thomas' Hospital & Guy's Hospital, London.
Letting epidurals wear off doesn't mean fewer assisted deliveries – Phillips KC et al: 'Second stage of labour with or without extradural analgesia', *Anaesthesia*, 1983 (38). Chestnut DH: 'Continuous epidural infusion of 0.0625% bupivacaine 0.0002% fentanyl during second stage of labour', *Anaesthesiology*, 1990 (72). Datta S: *Childbirth & Pain Relief*, Next Decade Publ, 2001.
Epidurals and backache: Kitzinger S: *Some Women's Experiences of Epidurals*,

The National Childbirth Trust, London, 1987. McArthur C, Lewis M et al: 'Epidural anaesthesia and long term backache after childbirth', *BMJ*, 1990 (301). McArthur C, Lewis M et al: 'Investigation of long term problems after obstetric epidural anaesthesia', *BMJ*, 1992 (304). Russell R, Groves P et al: 'Assessing long term backache after childbirth', *BMJ*, 1993 (306). McLeod J, Macintyre C et al: 'Backache and epidural anaesthesia', *Int J Obst Anaesth*, 1995. Breen TW, Ransil BJ: 'Factors associated with back pain after childbirth', *Anaesthesiology*, 1994 (81). Patel M, Fernando R: 'A prospective study of long term backache after childbirth in primigavidae – effect of ambulatory epidural anaesthesia', *Int J Obst Anaesth*, 1995, 4. Loughanan BA, Carli F et al: 'The influence of epidural anaesthesia on new backache', *Int J Obst Anaesth*, 1997 (6). *Regional Anaesthesia in Obstetrics – a Millennium Update*, Ed: Reynolds F, Springer, 2001.
Epidurals and Caesareans – Ramin SM, Grambling DR, Lucas MJ: 'Randomized trial of epidurals vs intravenous anaesthesia during labour', 13,350 women in the trial, *Obst Gyn*, 1996, 86. Thorpe: *Birth*, 2/6/1996 (23). Ramin SM, UT Southwestern Medical Centre, 869 women in trial, *Obst Gyn*, Nov 1995. Rydhstroem H, Central Hospital, Helsingbourg, Sweden: 'Combining Epidural Anaesthesia with Opioids Decreases Caesarean Risk'; 'Epidural anaesthesia with sufentanil during labour and operative delivery', *Acta Obstetrica et Gynecologica Scandanavia*, 2000 (79).

Caesareans

Caesareans and physicians – Goyert GL et al: 'The physician factor in Caesarean birth rates', *N Engl J Med*, 1989 (320). Neuhoff D et al: 'Caesarean birth for failed progress in labour', *Obst Gyn*, 1989 (73). Being conscious under GA – Scott DB: *Anaesthesia*, 46, p674. See also 'Epidurals and Caesareans' in Epidural section.

Pethidine

Not such a good pain-reliever for labour – Ranta P, Joupilla P, Spalding M et al: 'Patients' assessment of water blocks, pethidine, nitrous oxide, paracervical and epidural blocks in labour', *Int J Obst Anaesth*, 1994 (3). Oflofsson, Ekblom et al: 'Lack of analgesic effect or systematically administered morphine or pethidine on labour', *Br J Obst Gyn*, 1996, 103. 'Use of Regional Analgesia', *Regional Analgesia in Obstetrics*, Ed: Reynolds F, Springer, 2001.

Complementary Therapies – general

No. of trainee GPs wishing to train in a compl therapy – survey by Royal College of GPs, 1996/7.

Number of midwives using compl therapies: Tiran D: *Complementary Therapies for Pregnancy and Childbirth*, Balliere Tindall, 1999 (survey conducted in Leicestershire, 1997).

UK/US compl therapy usage figs – 'Complementary Therapies' and 'Holistic Medicine', *Reader's Digest Complete A-Z of Family Medicine & Health*, 2002. Consumers' Association: readership survey of usage, *Which*, 1996. The Institute of Complementary Medicine, UK, 2002.

Acupuncture

West Z: *Acupuncture in Pregnancy & Childbirth*, Churchill Livingstone, 2000. Yelland S, Acupuncture in Midwifery, *BFM*, 1986. Skelton I: *Acupuncture in Labour*, PhD thesis, publ by Royal College of Midwives, 1985. Yelland S: 'Using acupuncture in midwifery care', *Modern Midwife*, 5/1/1995.

Studies on acupuncture to relieve labour pain – Nilsson M: 'Acupuncture for Analgesia in Childbirth', *Jordmorbladet*, Jul-Aug 1993 (106). Cypriot trial: Martoudis & Christofides, 1990. Zeisler H, Temfer C et al, Univ Vienna: 'Influence of Acupuncture on Duration of Labour', *Gyn Obst Invest*, 1998 (46). Univ Hospital, Malmo, Sweden: 'Acupuncture for Pain Relief During Childbirth', *Acupunct Electrother Res*, 1998 (vol 23, 1). Tempfer C et al, Univ Vienna: 'Influence of Acupuncture on Maternal Serum Levels of interleukin-8, prostaglandin F2 alpha and beta endorphin: a matched pair study', *Obst Gyn*, Aug 1998 (vol 92). Kvorning, Ternov et al: 'Acupuncture during childbirth reduces the use of conventional analgesia without major side effects: a retrospective study', *Amer J Acupn*, 1998 (26). White AR: 'Acupuncture may help those who choose it in childbirth', *Alt Compl Th*, June 1999.

Speeding up labour – Ricci L: 'Agopuntura per l'induzione e l'analgesia nel travaglio di parto' (Acupuncture for induction and analgesia in childbirth), *Giornale Ital Rifflessoter Agopunt*, 1997.

Aromatherapy

General study of 8085 women using aromatherapy in labour in Oxford – Burns E, Blamey C et al: 'An investigation into the use of aromatherapy in intrapartum midwifery practice', *J Alt Compl Med*, 6/4/2000.

Clary sage for encouraging contractions, and lavender baths for pain –

Burns E and Blamey D: 'Using aromatherapy in childbirth', *Nursing Times*, 90 (9), 1994.
Clove oil for encouraging uterine contractions – Cutter K: 'Dedicated to better birth', *Int J of Aroma*, 4 (1) 11, 1992.
Lavender after childbirth to help sore perineum and encourage healing – Dale A, Cornwall S: 'The role of lavender oil in relieving perineal discomfort following childbirth: a blind, randomized clinical trial', *J Adv Nurs*, Jan 1994. Tiran D: *Clinical Aromatherapy for Pregnancy & Childbirth*, 2nd ed, Churchill Livingstone, 1999.

Autogenic Training

Schultz JH: *Autogenic Therapy, Vol ll*: Medical Applications, Grune & Stratton, New York/London, 1969. Yang I, Chin I, Chen W: 'The effect of EMG feedback and autogenic training in relieving the anxiety of pregnant women', *Acta Psychologica Sinica*, 4, 420, 1987. Kanji N: 'Management of Pain Through Autogenic Training', *Comp Th in Nursing & Midwifery*, 2000, 6, 143. Setter F, Kupper S: 'Autgenes Training – Qualitive Meta-Analyse kontrollierter klinischer Studien und Beziehungen zur Naturheilkunde', *Research in Complementary Medicine*, 1998, 5, 211. Lidnen W: 'Autogenic training: a narrative and quantitive review of clinical outcome', Dept Psych, Univ British Columbia, Canada: *Biofeedback Self Regul* 1994 Sept. Cattani P, Sin a P et al: 'Effect of autogenic respiratory training on labour pain', Inst Clinica Ostetrica e Ginelogica, Univ degli Studi di Verona, *Minerva Ginecol*, Nov 1991. De Punzio C, Neri E et al: 'The relationship between maternal relaxation and plasma beta endorphin levels during parturation', Dept Gyn e Ostetrica, Univ Pisa, Italy, *Psychosom Obst Gyn*, Dec 1994.

Breathing

Pugh LC et al: 'First stage labour management: an examination of patterned breathing and fatigue', *Birth*, 25/12/1998 (4).

Doulas

Case Western Reserve Univ School of Medicine, Ohio USA: 'Doula Support reduces Complications and Shortens Labour', *Pain Weekly*, 17/51999.
Banyana CM, Sandall J, McLeod C et al: 'Effects of Female Relative Support in Labour: A Randomized Controlled Trial', *Birth*, 1/3/1999 (26).
Kennell J, Klaus M et al: 'Continuous Emotional Support During Labour in a US Hospital', *JAMA*, 1/5/1991. Sosa, Kennell et al: 'The effects of a

supportive companion on perinatal problems, length of labour and mother-infant interaction', *New Eng J Med*, 1980 (303).

Men and doulas – Bertsch TD, Nagashima-Whalen L et al: 'Labour Support by First Time Fathers: Direct Observations', *J Psychosom Obst & Gyn*, 1990 (11). Chun Chi College Dept Nursing, Chinese Univ of Hong Kong: 'Relationships between partner's support during labour and maternal outcomes', *J Clin Nurs*, 9/3/2000 (2).

Homeopathy

Banerji P, Mukherjee S: *Standardisation of Treatment in Labour & Delivery*, proceedings from Indian conference report, 49th LMHI Congress, 1995, New Delhi.

Caulophyllum for non-progressing labour/rigid cervix/helping labour go smoothly – 'Applicability of Homeopathic Caulophyllum during labour', *Brit Homeo J*, Oct 1993 (82). Ventoskovskiy BM, Popov AV: 'Homeopathy as a practical alternative to traditional obstetric methods', *Brit Homeo J*, Oct 1990 (79). Brennan P: 'Homeopathic remedies in prenatal care', section on induction of labour, *J of Nursing & Midwifery*, May/June 1999 (44).

Volker Steckelbroeck MD, Hubner F, Klein P: 'Medication for Women with Rigid Uterine Cervix: a comparative examination', survey in Bruhl, *Biomedical Therapy*, 2000 (No 2). Gerber, R (MD): *Vibrational medicine for the 21st century*, Piatkus, 2000.

Bach Flower Remedies – recommendations from Howard J, midwife and senior Bach Flower Remedy tutor and author.

Hypnotherapy

General/shortening labour and pain relief – Connelly D: 'A comparison in drug usage between mothers who have trained in self-hypnosis and those who have no hypnosis training', presentation to the Irish Branch of the British Society of Experimental and Clinical Hypnosis, Belfast, 1989.

Harmon T, Hynan M, 'Improved obstetric outcomes using hypnotic analgesia and skill mastery combined with childbirth education', *J of Coun & Clin Psych*, 58, 5, 1990. Jenkins M, Pritchard M: 'Hypnosis: practical applications and theoretical considerations in normal labour', *Brit J Obst & Gyn*, 100, 221, 1990. Mairs D: 'Hypnosis and pain in childbirth', *Contemp Hypn*, 12, 2, 1995.

Suggestion therapy – Hao TY, Li YH: 'Clinical study on shortening the birth process using psychological suggestion therapy', Gen Military Hospital of Jinan, *Zonghua Hu Li Za Zhi*, Oct 1997 (32).

Turning breech babies – Mehl L: 'Hypnosis and conversion of breech to vertex presentation', *Archives of Family Medicine*, 3, 10, 1994.
Preventing premature birth – Omar H, Friedlander D: 'Hypnotic relaxation in the treatment of premature labour', *Psychsom Med*, 48, 5, 351, 1986.

Reflexology
Feder E, Liisberg GB et al: 'Zone therapy in relation to birth', proceedings of International Confederation of Midwives 23rd International Congress 2 (p 651-656), 1993. Motha G, McGrath J: 'The effects of reflexology on labour outcome', *J of Ass of Reflex*, 2-4, 1993.
Reflexology reducing pain in first stage of labour – Koraeva, Poluianova & Ustonova: Anesteziol Reanimatol, 1980. Tiran D: 'Reflexology in Midwifery Practice', *Complementary Therapies for Pregnancy & Childbirth*, Balliere Tindall, 1999.
Reflexology and light anaesthesia for Caesarean – Drs Zharkin, Frolov and Kostenko, *Akush Geinkol Mosk*, 1984. Zolnikov, Lapik, Ustonova and Shatkina: 'Reflexology in the Obstetric Clinic', overview article, *Akush Ginekol Mosk*, 1981. 'Zone reflex therapy for mothers', *Nursing Times*, 1990.

TENS
Approx 70-80% effective – Kaplan AU, Rabinerson D: 'Transcutaneous electrical nerve stimulation for adjuvant pain relief during labour and delivery', *Int J Gyn & Obst*, March 1998 (vol 60). Tischendorf D: 'Transcutaneous electrical nerve stimulation (TENS) in obstetrics', *Zentralbl Gynakol*, 1986 (108, 8).
Rise in endorphins with TENS: Lechner W et al: 'Beta endorphins during childbirth under TENS', *Zentralb Gynakol*, 1991, 113 (8).
TENS not much use – Van der Ploeg JM, Vervest HA et al: 'TENS during the first stage of labour: a randomised clinical trial', *Pain*, Nov 1996. Lee EW, Chung IW et al: 'The role of TENS in management of labour in obstetric patients', *Asia Oceania J Obst Gyn*, Sept 1990. Thomas IL, Tyle V et al: 'An evaluation of TENS for pain relief in labour', *Austr NZ J Obst Gyn*, Aug 1988.

Water
Beake S: 'Waterbirth: A Literature Review', *Practicing Midwife*, Feb 2000 (vol 3, no 2). Nikodem VC: 'Immersion in water during pregnancy, labour and birth', The Cochrane Library, Oxford, 1998. Jessman WC, Byers H:

'The Highland Experience: immersion in water in labour', *Brit J Midwifery*, June 2000.
Labour & birth in water as safe as on land for low-risk mothers, even if waters have broken – Randomised controlled trial of 1237 women, 'To study possible detrimental maternal and neonatal effects of immersion in warm water during labour', *Acta Obstetrica et Gynecologica Scandinavia*, April 2002 (80). Brown L: 'The Tide Has Turned: audit of waterbirth', *Brit J of Midwifery*, April 1998 (vol 6). Eriksson AV, Lanfors L et al: 'Warm tub bath during labour. A study of 1385 women with pre labour rupture of membranes after 34 weeks gestation', *Acta Obstetrica et Gynecologica Scandinavia*, 1996 4 (75). Garland D, Jones K: 'Waterbirth: Updating the evidence', *Brit J of Midwifery*, 1997 5 (6). Dept of Epidemiology & Public Health (Institute of Child Health, London): 'Perinatal mortality and morbidity among babies delivered in water', *BMJ*, 21/8/1999.
When to get in the pool – Hartley J: 'The use of water during labour and birth', *RCM Midwives' J*, Dec 1998 (1). Eriksson M, Mattsson LA: 'Early or late bath during the first stage of labour – a randomised study', *Midwifery*, Sept 1997 (vol 13, no 3).
Fewer perineal tears/episiotomies – Garland D, Jones K: 'Waterbirth: Updating the evidence', *Brit J of Midwifery*, 1997 5 (6). Geissbuhler V, Eberhard J: 'Waterbirths: a prospective study on more than 2000 waterbirths', *Fetal Diag Ther*, Sept/Oct 2000.

Water Injections

Oden M: 'Lumbar reflexotherapie: effective in the treatment of acute kidney pains and in obstetric analgesia', *La Nouvelle Presse Medicale*, Lettres, 1975 (4, no. 3). Martinson L: randomised controlled clinical trial at Dept Health Sciences, Univ of Skovode, Sweden, *Brit J Obst & Gyn*, July 1999.
Reynolds JL: 'Intracutaneous sterile water for back pain in labour', *Can Fam Physc*, Oct 1994. Labrecque M, Nouwen A et al: 'A randomised controlled trial on non-pharmacologic approaches for relief of low back pain during labour', Laval Univ, Sainte-Foy, Quebec, *J Fam Pract*, April 1999 (48, 4). Tandberg A: 'Intracutaneous injections of sterile water as analgesia during labour', *Tidsskr Nor Laegeforen*, 10/8/1990. Adler L, Hansson B: 'Parturition pain treated by intracutaneous injections of sterile water', *Pain*, 4/5/1990.

Resources

Contact the following for information on finding qualified complementary therapists, and teachers of/equipment for natural labour and birth techniques.

If you cannot find a therapist in your area, or need some general information, contact the **Institute of Complementary Medicine**, tel 020 7237 5165. It has a register of professional therapists of all types all over the country and can provide information on the therapies concerned.

Acupuncture
The British Acupuncture Council, tel 020 8735 0400 (see also Shiatsu). Sessions cost £25-£60 for the first one, less thereafter.

Aromatherapy
The Aromatherapy Organisations Council, tel 020 8251 7912. To get good quality oils, look out for Fragrant Earth and Tisserand brands. Also try Neal's Yard

Remedies rapid mail-order line, 0161 831 7875. Visit www.fleur.co.uk for a wide range of aromatherapy products, including factsheets on health and safety issues. Oils cost from £4 for 10ml of Lavender to £40 or more for Rose. Aromatherapy massage sessions cost approx £25-£45 for an hour or more.

Autogenic training

The British Society for Autogenic Training, tel 01923 675501. Classes cost about £150 for eight group sessions.

Bach Flower Remedies

The Dr Edward Bach Centre, tel 01491 834 678. Remedies cost £3-£4 for 10ml.

Birthing pools

These companies hire out portable birthing pools for you to use in hospital or at home, and will deliver and collect afterwards in most areas (people usually hire them for a couple of weeks as few babies arrive on their due date): the Active Birth Centre, London, tel 020 7482 5554 (prices from £110 p/w, with small charge per day after that); Splashdown, tel 020 8422 9308.

Breathing techniques and natural childbirth

The Active Birth Centre and The National Childbirth Trust (NCT), see below.

Doulas

For information log on to www.doula.freeserve.co.uk. To find one in your area write to Doula UK, PO Box 33817, London N8 9AW, or contact Top Notch Doulas, London, tel 020 7244 6053 (www.topnotchnannies.com/main.html).

Homeopathy

To find a medically qualified homeopath: The British Homeopathic Association, tel 020 7935 2163. For a lay

homeopath: The Society of Homeopaths, tel 0870
7703214. For good-quality homeopathic remedies by
mail order (24-48hrs delivery time): Helios
Homeopathic Pharmacy, Tunbridge Wells, tel 01892
537 254; Ainsworths Homeopathic Pharmacy, London,
tel 020 7935 5330.

Hypnotherapy and self-hypnosis
The College of Hypnotherapists & Psychotherapists has
the National Register of Hypnotherapists &
Psychotherapists, tel 01282 699 378 (all members are
psychotherapists qualified in hypnotherapy). British
Society of Medical and Dental Hypnosis, tel 07000
560309, or visit www.bsmdh.org. Hypnotherapy
sessions and teaching sessions cost £40-£70 for the
first one, less thereafter, and usually last one to
one-and-a-half hours.

Massage
Natural/active childbirth classes will usually teach some
massage as part of their course. If you have an
Independent Midwife Association (IMA) midwife she
will be able to show your partner special massage
techniques to use on you as well as being able to use
massage for labour on you herself. Massage sessions
from a masseur cost £20-£50 for an hour.

Reflexology
The Association of Reflexologists, tel 0870 567 3320.

Relaxation, visualisation and meditation techniques
These will be taught in Active Birth Centre antenatal
classes and by The National Childbirth Trust (NCT)
tutors countrywide, and briefly in NHS antenatal
classes. They are also taught in yoga classes: British
Wheel of Yoga, tel 01529 306851; TM (Transcendental
Meditation) UK, tel 08705 143733. They also form
part of Buddhist meditation classes: try The Friends of
the Western Buddhist Order, tel 020 8981 1225.

Classes cost £3-£7 and usually last one-and-a-half to two hours.

Shiatsu

The Shiatsu Society (www.shiatsu.org) is the official umbrella body for all types of shiatsu ('acupuncture without the needles') in the UK, tel 01788 555051. Sessions cost £25-£50 for the first one, less thereafter.

TENS

Several companies sell TENS machines but it is cheaper to hire one: try Abbey TeNS, Milton Keynes, tel 0845 1232605; Mothercare's TENS rental service, tel 01923 240365: and larger branches of Boots. Prices from about £25 for 4-5 weeks.

Back problems

The British Chiropractic Association

Tel 01189 505950. Specialists in back, neck and musculo skeletal problems. Sessions cost £30-£50 for the first one, less thereafter.

British School of Osteopathy (BSO)

Tel 020 7407 0222. Specialists in back, neck and musculo skeletal problems. Osteopaths have a different way of treating patients to chiropractors. The BSO holds a national register of all qualified osteopaths who trained with them. Sessions cost £30-£50 for the first one, less thereafter.

General help and support

Active Birth Centre

Tel 020 7482 5554. Runs fee-paying courses countrywide on natural and active childbirth techniques and yoga-for-pregnancy classes. It also offers support and advice to women who want to try for a natural childbirth or use water for any part of their labour. It hires out portable pools and can tell you which NHS hospitals offer them for women in labour, too. It has a wide range of pregnancy- and birth-related products and literature.

Association for Improvements in the Maternity Services (AIMS)
Helpline: 0870 7651433. Offers information and advice on all aspects of your maternity rights and options.

Caesarean Support Network
Tel 01624 661269 (evenings and weekends). Or write to the Caesarean Support Network, c/o 55 Cooil Drive, Douglas, Isle of Man IM1Y 2HF. Information, support and advice on all aspects of having a Caesarean, including the procedure itself, recovery, breastfeeding and future births.

Independent Midwives Association (IMA)
Tel 01483 821104. Or try writing to: IMA, 1 The Great Quarry, Guildford, Surrey GU1 3XN. Professional midwives who used to work in the NHS but now have their own private practices. Sympathetic to natural childbirth/active childbirth practices, including natural methods of pain relief such as water. Some are also trained in reflexology, homeopathy and acupuncture for childbirth. IMA members care for you throughout your pregnancy and labour and after the birth. They also do home births (they will transfer you to hospital and go with you should it become necessary). Fee scale from £1000-£4000, depending on where you live.

National Childbirth Trust (NCT)
Tel 020 8992 8637. Comprehensive information and support on every aspect of pregnancy, labour, birth and breastfeeding. There are NCT counsellors countrywide.

It also offers a wide range of pregnancy-, birth- and breastfeeding-related products and literature.

Royal College of Midwives (RCM)

Tel 020 7312 3535. Can advise you on all aspects of midwifery practice in the UK. It has information on the departments of midwifery in hospitals countrywide that are sympathetic to different ways of giving birth and natural forms of pain relief. If your hospital is not keen on your choice of pain relief, the RCM can advise you.

Twins and Multiple Births Association (TAMBA)

Tel 0870 770 3305. Or try writing to: TAMBA, 2 The Willows, Gardner Road, Guildford, Surrey GU1 4PG. Advice, information and support for parents of twins, triplets and more.

Glossary

Acupuncture An ancient Chinese form of medicine in which the tips of fine needles are inserted into specific parts of the body to treat illness and soothe pain.

Adrenaline A hormone produced by the adrenal gland in response to stress.

Alternative medicine The treatment, alleviation or prevention of illnesses using methods other than those used in conventional medicine.

Anaesthesia The loss of consciousness induced by drugs.

Anaesthetic Medication that causes loss of sensation, either to the whole body (general), in which case loss of consciousness is also produced, or a part of it (local).

Analgesia The medical term for pain relief. It may be a drug or a natural method.

Apgar score All newborns undergo a series of five checks to assess their overall wellbeing. Each check is given an 'Apgar' score of between zero and two.

Aromatherapy The use of essential oils of plants, thought to encourage the release of various neurochemicals in the body for pain-relieving, relaxing and healing purposes.

Assisted delivery Where medical intervention is needed to help the baby out of the vagina, using either forceps or a ventouse.

Auricular therapy A form of acupuncture in which needles are inserted into the ear only.

Autogenic training Deep relaxation therapy for relieving stress, which can be used to ease pain in labour.

Birth canal The unified passage of the womb, the dilated cervix and the vagina, along which a baby passes before being born.

Birthing pool A special warm water pool which provides pain relief to women in labour. It is much bigger than a bath and can accommodate at least two people.

Bradykinin An enzyme made in body tissues during muscle damage that irritates the nerve endings.

Braxton Hicks contractions During pregnancy the womb makes mild contractions as a way of limbering up and getting ready for labour. These are felt to different degrees, sometimes not at all, but they are not labour contractions and do not cause the cervix to dilate.

Breathing and relaxation A natural form of deep relaxation used for pain relief in labour. You need to practise it as often as possible prior to the birth to get the best effect.

Breech delivery When the baby is born bottom-first rather than head-first. A breech delivery is more difficult to manage and demands greater skill from the midwife and medical staff.

Caesarean section Delivery of the baby via an incision in the mother's abdomen and womb. It can be done under general anaesthetic, but is more usually done with an epidural or spinal.

Catecholamines Hormones that cause contractions of the womb and also act as pain transmitters. They are usually secreted in the second stage of labour, and encourage the strong, expulsive contractions of the womb that are needed at this time.

Cephalo-pelvic disproportion When the baby's head is too large to pass easily through the mother's pelvis. It may be because the baby has a very big head, because the head is incorrectly positioned, or because the mother has a smaller than average pelvis.

Cervix The neck, or exit, of the womb. In women who aren't pregnant it is almost closed, with an opening just a millimetre or two wide, through which menstrual blood escapes each month. Once pregnancy starts, it stays closed to keep the baby in the womb. During labour it dilates to 10cm to allow the baby out.

Complementary medicine The treatment, alleviation or prevention of illnesses using methods that are not practised in conventional medicine but are compatible with conventional medicine, eg acupuncture.

Contractions The clenching and flexing of the womb muscles in labour as they work to dilate the cervix, shrink the womb and push the baby down the birth canal.

Cortisol A hormone produced by the adrenal gland that helps the body cope with psychological and physiological stress.

Doula A woman with positive experiences of childbirth and a good basic knowledge of it, who stays with and supports a mother during her labour. She usually helps the mother for the first few days or weeks after the baby has been born, too.

Distraction therapy Using an activity to distract yourself from registering pain – for example, watching a music video as a dentist is drilling your tooth, or practising controlled breathing while in early labour.

Dura The membranes that form the sac containing the spinal fluid, the spinal cord and its nerves.

Eclampsia The severe form of pre-eclampsia (see Pre-eclampsia), which can affect pregnant women. Symptoms include very high blood pressure, convulsions and headaches. It is an extremely rare condition, as the symptoms of pre-eclampsia are nearly always picked up and treated immediately.

Elective Caesarean A Caesarean section that has been planned well in advance.

Endorphins Powerful morphine-like hormones produced by the body that help kill pain and lift a person's mood.

Entonox A form of pain relief, often called gas and air, consisting of a mixture of nitrous oxide and oxygen that the mother breathes in during contractions.

Epidural The most effective medical technique for relieving labour pain. A powerful local anaesthetic drug is injected into the tissues around the spinal sac to numb the nerves. The mother loses most of the feeling below her waist. Different from a spinal anaesthetic.

Episiotomy A surgical cut made under local anaesthesia in the perineum to enlarge the vagina's exit to make more room for the baby's head.

False labour When Braxton Hicks contractions are so strong and regular that they are mistaken for real labour contractions, or when labour seems to begin but then dies away.

Fetal distress This is when the unborn baby becomes short of oxygen. It can be dangerous, and is one of the major reasons why a mother has to have a Caesarean section.

Fetal medicine The science of understanding and looking after unborn babies.

Fetus The medical term for a baby in the womb from eight weeks until birth.

First stage of labour When the womb is contracting and the neck of it, the cervix, is opening. By the end of the first stage the cervix has opened up completely to about 10cm wide.

Forceps A surgical instrument sometimes used in assisted deliveries to ease the baby out of the vagina. It looks a little like a pair of metal salad servers.

Gas In terms of pain relief this usually refers to nitrous oxide (sometimes called laughing gas). See Entonox.

General anaesthetic A combination of drugs that produces loss of feeling in the entire body, with loss of consciousness. Women having emergency Caesareans will often have one for their operation.

Homeopathy A method of treating a wide range of conditions by the use of tiny amounts of natural substances diluted many thousands of times. If given in large quantities, the remedies produce symptoms similar to those of the illness being treated.

Hormone A chemical substance carried in the blood to tissues, on which it exerts a specific effect.

Hypnotherapy The use of hypnosis to treat a wide range of problems, including labour pain.

Induction A procedure to start labour artificially. A mother might be given prostaglandin pessaries or have her waters broken. Acupuncture can also be used.

Intravenous drip The continuous infusion of fluids directly into the bloodstream via a tube in a vein.

Ischaemia Lack of oxygenated blood to muscles. When a muscle becomes starved of oxygen it will spasm painfully. This is one cause of pain in labour.

Labour The process of childbirth. It is the time from when the womb begins to contract and the cervix to open, to the delivery of the placenta after the baby has been born.

Lactic acid An organic acid secreted as a waste product when muscle cells are working. It is usually broken down into carbon dioxide and breathed out through the lungs. If the muscles are working very hard, as in labour, the acid can build up and irritate the nerve endings running through the muscle fibres, causing pain.

Meconium The greenish waste substance that fills the large bowel of the fetus. Usually it stays there until after delivery, when it becomes that baby's first bowel movement. But if the fetus becomes short of oxygen, its large bowel may contract and push the meconium into the amniotic fluid that surrounds it. This then passes out of the vagina as a greenish watery substance at the entrance. The appearance of meconium during labour is one sign of fetal distress.

Mobile epidural A form of epidural (see Epidural) that enables the mother to change position freely and even walk about during labour.

Morphine A very powerful pain-relieving drug derived from opium.

Narcotic Any drug that produces numbness and stupor and relieves pain.

Natural childbirth A method of childbirth in which the mother is left free to follow her own instincts for labour and birth (perhaps to move around, remain upright or semi-upright, and/or deliver her baby while squatting). She doesn't use any pain-relieving drugs or have any medical intervention.

Natural pain relief The reduction or elimination of pain using drug-free methods, such acupuncture and relaxation and breathing.

Nitrous oxide A gas that is usually mixed with oxygen and breathed in through the mouth. See also Entonox.

Oxytocin A hormone produced in the pituitary gland that stimulates the womb to contract. It *may* also produce partial amnesia about the labour for both mother and baby.

Pain threshold The point at which a stimulus is perceived as painful, whether it is heat from a flame or pain from a contraction. Most people's pain thresholds are similar – it is their tolerance levels that vary.

Pain tolerance The ability to endure pain. How high or low a person's pain tolerance is depends on how they cope with pain once it has exceeded the pain threshold. Using pain-relieving methods, whether natural or medical, will increase a person's pain tolerance.

Paracervical block Injection of a local anaesthetic to numb the nerves that run from the womb to either side of the cervix. If used, it is usually given at the end of the first stage of labour. It is useful for assisted deliveries but is rarely used in the UK, having been mostly replaced by epidurals.

Pelvic floor The sling of muscles within the pelvis that supports the bladder and womb.

Perinatal The period around birth, starting a few weeks before the birth and ending a couple of weeks afterwards.

Perineum This is the muscular area between the opening of the vagina and the rectum. It stretches considerably in front of the baby's head during birth.

Pethidine A pain-relieving and sedative drug.

Pharmacological pain relief Pain-killing drugs that can only be given to you by qualified medical or midwifery staff.

Placenta The organ that develops on the inner wall of the womb in pregnancy. It supplies the fetus with oxygen and nutrients and carries away waste products to the mother's system.

Placental abruption When the placenta begins to separate from the womb wall, causing considerable bleeding. This requires immediate action, often an emergency Caesarean.

Potency A measure of how strong a homeopathic medicine is. Different people have different responses to these remedies, and so may require a higher or lower potency to achieve the same effect.

Placenta praevia A condition in which the placenta is attached low down on the womb wall, possibly blocking or partially blocking the exit from the womb. This part of the womb stretches in the last few weeks of pregnancy, but because the placenta can't stretch with it, it becomes detached, causing bleeding that can often be severe. It is usually diagnosed well in advance of the birth with ultrasound, and the mother is advised about the safest method of delivery, usually a Caesarean.

Pre-eclampsia A condition that can affect pregnant women. Symptoms include high blood pressure, protein in urine, above average weight gain and fluid retention. It may affect the growth of the fetus, resulting in a small baby. It can often be controlled by rest, medication and diet, but may mean admission to hospital during the latter part of pregnancy and a medically managed labour or even a Caesarean. If it becomes severe it can lead to eclampsia.

Prenatal Before the baby is born.

Prostaglandins Hormone-like substances that help stimulate the onset of labour contractions.

Pudendal block An injection of local anaesthetic to block the nerves that supply the perineum, thereby numbing it during delivery. Also used for episiotomies.

Reflexology A therapy in which gentle pressure is applied to specific points on the hands and feet to help treat disorders, encourage relaxation, or reduce pain.

Sacrum Curved triangular part of the backbone at the base of the spine, comprising five fixed vertebrae.

Second stage of labour The part of childbirth when the mother pushes the baby out through the birth canal to be born.

Show The discharge of a little bloodstained mucus from the vagina. This is one of the signs of the onset of labour.

Spinal An injection of local anaesthetic into the fluid around the spinal cord. It usually provides total pain relief very fast. It is not the same as an epidural.

Tears During delivery small splits in the fleshy lips at the entrance to the vagina may occur. These may need stitching after the birth but usually heal quickly and easily on their own.

Third stage of labour The part of childbirth when, after the birth of the baby, the placenta is delivered.

Transcutaneous Electrical Nerve Stimulation (TENS) A form of pain relief involving a low-grade electrical current – passed through pads on the mother's back – that helps prevent pain signals from the womb reaching the brain.

Transition A phase at the end of the first stage of labour, immediately before the second, when the cervix finishes dilating to 10cm and the womb's contractions change to a different type that push the baby out.

Transverse lie When the baby is lying sideways in the womb, as opposed to head-down (the most usual position). It is sometimes possible to encourage the baby to turn into the correct position by manual manipulation and massage (your obstetrician should do this), and there have also been cases where acupuncture and homeopathy have worked. It is unlikely that a baby lying this way can be delivered vaginally – a Caesarean is usually necessary.

Ultrasound A method of examining unborn babies using sound waves to build an image of them on a computer screen.

Umbilical cord The cord that connects the unborn baby to the placenta.

Vacuum extraction Assisted delivery using a suction device.

Ventouse A surgical suction device that can be attached to the baby's head in assisted deliveries to ease him out of the vagina.

Visualisation Concentrating on 'seeing' something in the mind's eye in order to encourage it to happen in reality.

Water injections A simple, drug-free method of relieving bad back pain, which involves two injections of sterile water on either side of the base of the spine. The resulting collections of water press on nerves coming from the base of the spine, interrupting the pain signals that travel along them.

Water birth Birth of the baby under water.

Womb (uterus) A muscular organ in a woman's body that contains the growing baby. During the first stage of labour it contracts to make itself smaller and open the cervix. During the second stage of labour it changes the way it contracts to push the baby out to be born.

Vagina The canal between the womb and the external genitals through which the baby is born.

Index